The EVERYTHING® Massage Book

Dear Reader:

I am honored to be involved with your journey into the evolving wonders of touch through massage. The experience of giving and receiving massage is one that you will cherish and grow with. Once you have begun the exploration into massage, the possibilities are endless. Imagine entire families sharing in the gift of giving through loving and compassionate touch. We never outgrow the need to love and be loved—caring touch satisfies this need completely.

The joy of massage for me has been in the seeing and knowing that we can help someone to feel better, emotionally and physically. To touch is to heal; how blessed is that! My intention here is to share my years of experience and knowledge with you by creating an easy guide that encourages you to try massage on yourself and others.

Namaste,

Valerie Voner

The EVERYTHING® Series

Editorial

Publishing Director	Gary M. Krebs
Managing Editor	Kate McBride
Copy Chief	Laura MacLaughlin
Acquisitions Editor	Eric M. Hall
Development Editor	Christina MacDonald
Production Editor	Jamie Wielgus

Production

Production Director	Susan Beale
Production Manager	Michelle Roy Kelly
Series Designers	Daria Perreault
	Colleen Cunningham
Cover Design	Paul Beatrice
	Frank Rivera
Layout and Graphics	Colleen Cunningham
	Rachael Eiben
	Michelle Roy Kelly
	John Paulhus
	Daria Perreault
	Erin Ring
Series Cover Artist	Barry Littmann
Interior Photography	Jonathan Allain Photography

Visit the entire Everything® Series at www.everything.com

THE
EVERYTHING®
MASSAGE
BOOK

Practical, simple techniques you can use at home
to relieve stress, promote healing, and feel great

Valerie Voner, L.M.T., C.R.T., R.M.T.

Recommended by:

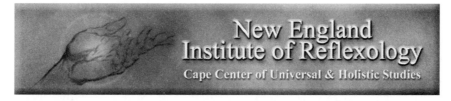

New England
Institute of Reflexology
Cape Center of Universal & Holistic Studies

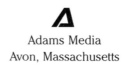

Adams Media
Avon, Massachusetts

To my entire family—you make my reality complete.

An Everything® Series Book.
Everything® and everything.com® are registered trademarks of F+W Publications, Inc.

Published by Adams Media, an F+W Publications Company
57 Littlefield Street, Avon, MA 02322 U.S.A.
www.adamsmedia.com

ISBN: 1-59337-071-7
Printed in the United States of America.

J   I   H   G   F   E   D   C   B   A

Library of Congress Cataloging-in-Publication Data
Voner, Valerie.
The everything massage book / Valerie Voner.
p.   cm.
(An everything series book.)
ISBN 1-59337-071-7
1. Massage. I. Title. II. Series: Everything series.
RA780.5.V66   2004
615.8'22–dc22   2004002187

*This book is available at quantity discounts for bulk purchases.
For information, call 1-800-872-5627.*

Contents

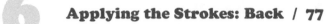

Acknowledgments

Thank you to every teacher I have encountered during my journey into the healing work of compassionate touch. I thank God for the many blessings I receive and for the opportunity to work in service. Thank you, Taylor, my son, for the support from you and your family, Jen, Ashley, and baby Taylor. Amber, thank you for allowing me to finish the book on your birthday; you are a great daughter. To all my siblings and my parents, much love. My agent Barb Doyen and my editor Eric Hall, to you I give thanks for always pushing and supporting through the tough times. Many blessings to my friends; your love and support sustained me. Thank you reader for choosing this book. May you enjoy massage as much as I do. In peace, namaste.

Top Ten
Benefits of Massage

1. Massage is kind and compassionate touch.

2. Massage allows for communication without words.

3. Massage helps to soothe heartburn, abdominal pain, and other stress-related digestive problems.

4. Chronic pain is lessened through regular massage.

5. Receiving massage during pregnancy helps ease back pain and supports muscle health.

6. A five-minute massage can ease and energize.

7. Regular massage encourages all the body systems to function properly.

8. Massage helps alleviate stress and sinus headaches while reducing tension in the neck.

9. Babies who receive massage cry less and are healthier.

10. Massage creates and promotes a strong feeling of connection between giver and receiver.

Introduction

▶FROM THE DAWN OF HUMANKIND, humans have recognized the importance and comfort of touch. Massage is the natural inclination to touch, to soothe, to rub, or to take away or ease whatever ails you. You are part of this rich history, contributing with your touch. Massage opens the door to discovery as your hands and fingers begin to see the aches and pains before you rub them away! A loving back rub becomes an experiment in touch as you travel through the variety of massage strokes to the joy of your partner. Massage is a tender gift you give as you gently stroke your baby's belly, watching as she kicks back in laughter.

Massage is a form of communication; you can actually talk to someone without words. When you are gently rubbing the tired arms and hands of a beloved elder you are expressing your feelings through the compassion of your touch. There is no mystery in this form of communication; this is open and honest giving. The energy between you and your receiver flows free and clear. Kind touch is about love.

Touch through massage is a sharing of self with others. A relationship of honor and trust is established through the give-and-take of caring touch. To receive massage is to trust the giver, to give massage is to honor the receiver. The knowledge you gather from this book will contribute to your relationship with yourself as well as with others. You are opening a door to whole wellness as you study educated touch, visualizing your hands as tools of healing. Massage takes away the aches and pains while providing comfort in the most basic of our instincts, touch.

Massage is used today in a variety of settings. It is used for everyone from athletes to infants to businessmen. Massage is used in physical therapy and in specific treatment of certain medical conditions. Massage has become popular in many areas of healing, including nursing and spa treatments, and is used by doctors for certain drugless healing.

This book is a how-to guide for learning to use massage and share its gifts. You will learn various techniques to use on yourself, as well as friends and family. You may even discover that you would like to pursue a career in massage, in which case the last chapter is a tool to assist you in finding the right school for you.

We discuss the different strokes and movements within a massage, and explore the variety of massages available, giving you an array of choices. As you develop an informed touch, your fingers will know what to do on the body you are massaging.

Through the study and examination of massage you will enter into a new world that is exciting and free. You will find that the physical and emotional relaxation you experience as a receiver and a giver frees your spirit. Welcome to the world of joyous giving. Feel free to jump in and try out your strokes.

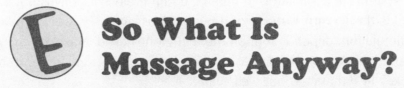

Chapter 1

So What Is Massage Anyway?

Anyone thinking about massage can usually conjure up a picture composed of one person relaxing and another person applying smooth, steady strokes to promote further relaxation. The body is the perfect palette for massage, the skin's surface calling for touch. In fact, your intuitive response to pain, whether physical or emotional, is to reach out and touch, instinctively rubbing the offending area and soothing your pain. Massage is simply an organized expression of your own natural ability.

Understanding What Massage Is

Massage is a system that promotes holistic health, which is the balance of body, mind, and spirit in a healthy, drug-free environment. We can describe massage as the manipulation of soft tissue and muscle in the support of natural healing, using hands, arms, and fingers as the tools. The systematic application of healing touch creates an environment of balance that in turn fosters good health. Massage may provide relaxation or stimulation, depending upon the techniques used. Massage encourages joy and happiness, whether as the receiver or the giver. In short, massage is a key to enhancing our well-being.

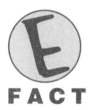

FACT

Our bodies have an innate gift—the capacity to promote our own healing. Touch is an effective tool in triggering this natural healing response. Massage enables the body to relax, creating a therapeutic environment for the healing functions of the body.

The Stimulation of the Senses

Our greatest sense receptor, the skin, is the obvious target in touch therapy, yet massage affects all of the senses. The use of warm scented oil on skin activates the sense of smell, further assisting in the area of relaxation. If the oil also has medicinal properties its natural healing abilities are stimulated, working the body toward greater balance. Receiving massage with our eyes closed allows us to mentally visualize the soothing effects—seeing through feeling. Hearing the soft calming music lulls us to an even deeper space of relaxation, allowing us to release all tension. The healing touch communicates with our brain, sending messages of trust, allowing the body to relax further.

Nerve and Tissue Response

Soft tissue responds to massage, releasing tension from tight muscles as well as supporting the flow of oxygen throughout the body. As the circulation of oxygen and blood is stabilized the body is encouraged to operate properly. Massage stimulates the nervous system by addressing the nerves directly under the skin as well as the main branches radiating from the spine.

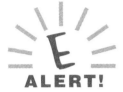

ALERT!

Pain is a natural signal alerting us to a malfunction within the body, an early warning not to be ignored. The pain response is present to sound the alarm, guiding us to seek the proper attention. Pain alerts us to begin the hunt to find the cause.

The nervous system speaks to every muscle and organ in the body. Because massage maintains nerve health, it supports whole health. As the connective tissue of the body is restored to high function through massage, the emotional self responds with a deeper sense of well-being. This feeling of peace spreads to a spiritual level as massage sustains the connection of body, mind, and spirit.

What Does Massage Do?

Massage creates a relaxed state of being. Regular sessions of massage significantly reduce our stress. Massage stimulates proper circulation, assisting the oxygen and blood to flow through the body correctly. Improper circulation can cause stiffness and cramping in a muscle. We all know what a toe or leg cramp feels like, especially in the middle of the night!

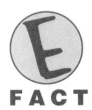

FACT

For years we have all been taught to stretch before and after exercise. Newer research reports that stretching a cold muscle is not the best practice. We need to gently warm up muscles and connective tissue first as further prevention from injury. Walking for five minutes or so before stretching is one of the best ways to relax and loosen stiff joints and muscles.

A congested muscle not only hinders body function but also represents an energy block. This block can create an area of distress that can lead to a chronic state of weakness. To prevent such blockages here are a few easy suggestions:

- Breathe, correctly, before, during, and after any form of exertion.
- Walk before you run.
- Stretch after any sustained exercise.
- Learn massage and use it.
- Practice simple yoga.
- Meditate regularly.
- Visualize yourself as strong and well.

Massage not only helps to maintain wellness, it also encourages the return of good health. Our bodies consist of cells that compose the tissue of bone, skin, muscle, tendons, ligaments, and fascia, as well as nerves, veins, and arteries. Many conditions respond to the healing touch of massage. Headaches lessen as the tissue of the head is relaxed, allowing the flow of oxygen and blood to feed the brain and surrounding nerves and muscles. Chronic pain is reduced, if not banished, by continued application of massage. Muscles relax, digestion improves, and the system of elimination responds to massage. Massage is a complement to any medical treatment, further supporting the treatment's healing effects.

The History of Massage

Massage has roots in every ancient culture. People everywhere from the beginning of time instinctively touched with kindness and love. To touch, to hold, to hug, to rub—these are inclinations that are universally owned. Even the earliest tribal cultures throughout the world included some form of massage when curing the sick. Tribal healers known as shamans served as priests as well as doctors, and physical healing was intertwined with spirit. Early shamanic practice involved rubbing the skin as a form of healing. The shamanic technique was to rub the skin from the center of the body out to the extremities, ridding the body of the disease and bad spirits by pushing out.

Eastern Massage Practices

The ancient Chinese developed the procedure of anma or anmo, a massage technique of pressing and rubbing particularly on specific areas to warm the extremities and heal the organs. Just as tribal cultures believed that body and spirit were not separate, so did the ancient Chinese, who believed if you heal one, you heal the other. Chinese massage was considered an important aspect of healing, and schools developed to teach the different methods.

Anmo massage from China was practiced in Japan and eventually developed into shiatsu. Built on the concept of balance within, shiatsu was and is used to improve all functions by applying finger pressure along the energy meridians (see Chapter 18 for more about shiatsu and meridians).

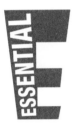

The improvement of Asian massage techniques continued with the advent of acupuncture, often combining it with shiatsu. Both shiatsu massage and acupuncture focus on the same points on the energy meridians of the body.

Although the first written mention of massage is found in China, travel between China, India, and Egypt suggests that each of these countries may have developed a style of massage unique to their individual cultures, although similar in some aspects. India is credited with a form of massage and bathing known as shampooing, a massage method that is still used today in Indian and Arabic cultures. The massage techniques were done in a steam-bath environment, and the strokes included kneading, tapping, friction, and joint manipulation.

Massage in Greece and Rome

The practices of massage and exercise flourished within ancient Greek society. The physician and priest Aesculapius was instrumental in the development of the famous Greek gymnasiums where the combination of massage, exercise, and water treatments was promoted to rid the body of disease and support whole health. Aesculapius was awarded the divine rank of god of medicine.

Hippocrates (c. 460–377 B.C.), known as the father of modern medicine, is also credited as a promoter of massage. Hippocrates' work was based on the idea that the body needs to be balanced to function properly. He prescribed massage as a tool to bring the body into wellness.

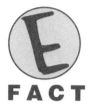

FACT

Hippocrates revolutionized the practice of medicine with his new ideas and new procedures. He introduced the concept of symptoms as they relate to the environment of the patient, using the symptoms as a guideline for treatment. Hippocrates was one of the first physicians to actually listen to the heart.

Hippocrates created a type of rubbing called anatripsis. The introduction of anatripsis revolutionized the practice of rubbing. Unlike the old shamanic style of massage, where the goal was to rub the evil spirits and illness out and away from the body, stroking toward the extremities, Hippocrates believed rubbing toward the heart to be more effective. He felt that massage moved the body fluids toward the center of the body, allowing for effective release of toxins and freeing the waste to leave the body.

The Roman era continued the support of massage and water therapy, using these treatment tools for chronic pain and muscle disorder, as well as for disease. Unlike the Greeks, the Romans instituted no formal training for physicians, and most doctors were under-trained slaves, barbers, or priests. Massage was often administered by slaves working in the gymnasiums. These massage providers could be called upon to practice medicine as well.

Claudius Galen (c. A.D. 129–216) was a prolific Greek writer and physician. Galen spent most of his years in Rome where he provided massage and bath therapy to the gladiators as well as to a number of Roman emperors. Galen wrote detailed instructions for exercise, massage, and water therapy that were treatments for specific injuries and ailments.

The decline of the Roman Empire brought unfortunate changes to the world of medicine, because many of the healthful practices were suppressed and forbidden. Although physicians and medical transcribers who lived through this long period of history still endorsed the use of massage, bathing, and exercise, these significant medical findings, along with other teachings, were nearly lost.

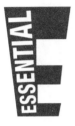

Julius Caesar, an epileptic, suffered also from neuralgia, a painful nerve condition that caused excruciating pain over areas of his body and head. He received friction-type massage as treatment for the neuralgia and prevention of epileptic episodes.

Arab Physicians Keep Massage Alive

As Europe declined, the Arab nations endorsed and utilized the teachings of Hippocrates and Galen, as well as the ancient philosophers of Greece and Rome. A Persian named Al-Kazi (A.D. 864–930), also known as Rhazes, was a great Muslim physician and a productive writer who was greatly influenced by these early beliefs and traditions. This supreme clinician could describe the clinical signs of many illnesses. With this awareness he would often recommend the use of diet, exercise, baths, and massage.

Another Persian physician, Ibn Sina, also known as Avicenna (A.D. 980–1037) was also heavily influenced by Roman and Greek medical practice. A copious writer, he is most famous for *The Canon of Medicine*. The *Canon* is a book that classifies, describes, and presents the causes of innumerable diseases. This book references massage and the use of baths and exercise as treatment of the classified diseases.

Massage During the Nineteenth Century

The natural treatment of disease using the ancient European healing concepts celebrated a renewal in the 1800s. Modern-day massage can trace its roots from this time period when prevention of disease and the upkeep of good health became the goals of medicine. The revival of physical exercise as a form of natural healing could be seen in all aspects of healing work from this time forward. Drugs and surgery as a way of healing were in use and some practitioners began to research the gymnasium experience as an alternative.

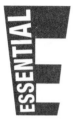

Modern medicine is built on allopathy, the use of drugs and surgeries to deal with the *effects* of the disease, but not the *cause*. Traditional medicine is homeopathic, meaning it treats the cause of the disease. Integration of the two styles gives you the best treatment.

In the early 1800s, Peter Ling, a Swedish physiologist and fencing master, adapted a system of exercise known as medical gymnastics. Along with active exercise and active-passive movements performed with the help of a therapist, Ling's system stressed the importance of passive movements. These entailed stroking, kneading, rubbing, friction, gliding, shaking, and many more movements that are clearly massage techniques.

Ling established the Royal Swedish Central Institute of Gymnastics, where the Swedish movements were studied. Schools flourished throughout Europe and training programs were developed to teach these healing techniques. Two American brothers, George and Madison Taylor, studied the Swedish movement and brought Ling's methods home to the States where they set up an orthopedic practice in New York.

Acceptance of the Terminology of Massage

Finally in the late 1800s the word *massage* was actually used to describe an individual healing component. Massage was considered its own modality with its own language. The terms "effleurage," "petrissage," "tapotement," and "massage" were used when speaking of the application of these techniques in conjunction with physical therapy. Books were published dealing with instruction in Swedish massage as well as other information provided by physicians who used massage as a form of healing.

Massage Today

Today massage is a viable profession that serves many purposes. A professional massage practitioner receives a structured training in a state-licensed school that deals solely with massage. Massage professionals have founded various organizations and associations that represent massage and other bodyworkers as well. For example, the National Certification Board for Therapeutic Massage and Bodywork imposes strict standards of practice and requires continuing evidence of competency, bringing the status of massage into the realm of professionalism in healthcare.

Massage has undeniable benefits that integrate well with other forms of treatment. Research has proven that massage improves circulation, including the movement of lymph, relieves congestion between joints, and helps to release tension and stress from the body. The history of massage is a rich tapestry woven with many brilliant colors and textures. The art of massage continues, because the tapestry is a work of art in progress. As you practice the techniques you learn here, you add your piece to the tapestry, weaving a pattern that is especially you.

Who Will Use Massage?

Anyone can benefit from massage, as a giver or a receiver. The natural instinct of a parent to rub a baby's back brings instant calmness and comfort to both the baby and the parent. We all reach out to touch another who is suffering from physical, emotional, or spiritual pain. A simple touch of the hand indicates empathy and compassion.

The specific use of massage is found in many arenas. Massage application is found in hospice, elder care, pregnancy, and childbirth. It is an important asset in health care today and may be found in chiropractors' offices, in association with physical therapy, and in hospitals as part of a recovery plan. Massage is equally important in the field of exercise, helping the athlete stay fit and pain free, and the beauty business endorses the use of massage as well.

Massage and Recovery

Studies indicate compassionate touch speeds recovery from illness, and provides a release from tension that hastens healing. Whether a person is in the hospital or at home, gentle massage will support the return to health. As the tissues are massaged, the muscles relax and take in oxygen and blood, which helps the body gather strength. The depletion felt following an illness is often lessened, at times even eliminated, through massage.

People afflicted with arthritis enjoy massage, finding relief from joint and connective tissue pain. The lack of mobility arthritis sufferers experience is often lessened with repeated massage. Arthritis, a degenerative joint disease, is one of many in this group of diseases sharing the commonality of inflammation, pain, and restricted movement of the joints. Massage is one of the ways to bring relief to those with these ailments.

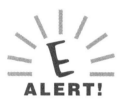

ALERT!

Massage is not indicated when arthritic joints are inflamed. The body is naturally protecting itself from further overuse by creating inflammation of joints, which results in stiffness, swelling, excess heat in the affected area, as well as aching. Wait until the swelling subsides before massaging the inflamed region.

Massage and Work

Standing on our feet for eight hours a day, whether as a waitress, a teacher, a builder, a nurse, or any other occupation that requires standing, puts great stress on the muscles of the back, legs, and neck. Those who must sit all day at their jobs cause harmful stress to other joints and muscles, such as back, hips, and shoulders, and inhibit natural circulation. The danger of tension coupled with muscle strain or lack of circulation needs to be reduced. Frequent massage is essential for the health and well-being of all our muscles when the body is stressed from constant standing or sitting.

Folks who work with repetitive motion benefit from massage, too. Whether wielding a hammer or typing on a keyboard, constant use of the same muscles within the body structure often weakens the muscles in the surrounding area as well as those doing the work. People in service to others, such as medical professionals, emergency workers, educators, parents, and bodyworkers, call on their bodies to perform often with no regard to rest. For those people, receiving massage is receiving instruction on relaxation. The person being worked on will surrender, releasing the mind and the body to calmness.

Massage and Sports

Massage is a useful tool in the overall conditioning of muscles used for action in exercise. By stimulating muscles, massage tones them for peak performance. Massaging the muscles after strenuous exercise also helps to relax them, pulling out waste quickly. If an injury has been sustained, massage improves circulation and lymphatic function allowing for speedier repair.

Don't Forget Your Pet

Animals love massage, too. Dogs and horses in particular will allow us to gently, yet firmly stroke with steady even pressure along their muscles. A young pet learns to relax and receive, creating a pattern that can continue throughout the life of the animal. Cats, too, will allow massage, generally for a shorter period of time. Whatever pet you have, try gently stroking along the back or legs, introducing this form of touch slowly. Massage helps a nervous animal relax and creates an atmosphere of quiet tranquility.

Can I Learn Massage Myself?

Anyone can learn to massage—all it takes is the desire to learn compassionate touch. We all know how to touch with care; the next step is to discipline that knowledge into an effective system of massage. Massage is fun and a source of pleasure and tenderness. Whether you massage yourself, a friend, or a loved one, the therapeutic art of massage brings awareness of the body to the forefront in you and the recipient.

Relaxation and Massage

We have briefly discussed muscle awareness and how to recognize release of tension. The act of giving a massage is an instruction in total relaxation. Initial contact wordlessly educates the body to trust another and ourselves and to create an environment of healing. Every position silently focuses the recipient on letting go, reminding the muscles to release, relax, and restore.

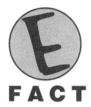

FACT

Many of us do not use our lungs to their full capacity; rather, we take short, shallow breaths. Inhale deeply through your nose, feeling the breath fill your diaphragm. Hold the breath, then slowly exhale, feeling the abdomen contract, pushing the air out. As we learn to breathe properly, we feel more relaxed, yet energized.

If you try this simple exercise in muscle relaxation yourself, you can begin to experience the process of body awareness that is so important in massage. Sit in a comfortable chair, your feet flat on the floor with your hands resting either on the arms of the chair or at your side. If you prefer, lie flat on a mat, hands by your sides. Close your eyes and become comfortable with your breath:

1. Breathe in slowly, letting your breath fill deep into your stomach.
2. Hold your breath in for a count of three and gently exhale, feeling all the air releasing.
3. Inhale again, becoming aware of your hands; they may begin to tingle or feel heavy.
4. As you exhale, stay connected to your hands.
5. Once more, breathe in deeply and hold your breath, feeling your belly push out.
6. Slowly let the air leave you again, flattening your abdomen.
7. Gently shake your hands, feeling all tension begin to leave your body.
8. Relax your feet, letting each bone, muscle, tendon, and ligament relax and sinking down to rest.
9. Move up to your calf and shin areas and relax them.

10. Feel your feet and lower legs become heavy, letting go of any hidden pockets of tension.
11. Bring your awareness to your knees, let them relax, sinking down into the ground. Feel your thighs and hamstrings relax.
12. Release the last remnants of tension from your hips and buttocks, letting yourself completely rest the lower part of your body.
13. Feel your back relax; let your spine sink down and relax; imagine every nerve and muscle in your back completely at rest.
14. Let your shoulders relax now and your arms; begin to feel every part of your hands from your wrist to your fingers; relax.
15. As you gently breathe in and out, every organ is relaxing, slowing down, as a sense of calmness permeates within; try to feel that calmness.
16. Now move up to your neck, letting all the muscles here relax.
17. Feel your face relax, your jaw, mouth, tongue, and teeth; let your cheeks relax as well as your sinuses and your nose; let your eyes and forehead relax.
18. Imagine a small glowing light appearing behind your eyelids, between your eyebrows in the center of your forehead; this is your third eye, your psychic center.
19. Imagine this light and let it flow up to the top of your head and down the back of your body, following the spine and then the nerves, down to your soles. Color the light with a soft glow of pink or opal.
20. Feel yourself completely relaxed, every part of you free from tension and worry. This is the feeling we achieve when we experience massage. It is with this intention that we enter into a relationship with touch therapy.

Compassionate touch through massage heals on all levels. It helps us to relax, which in turn feeds the body, the mind, and the soul. It develops in us a sense of trust so that we can give massage as well as receive it. Giving and receiving massage develops a profound sense of self.

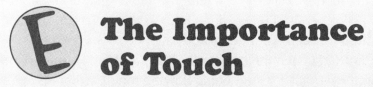

Chapter 2

The Importance of Touch

In massage, your eyes often reside in your fingers and hands, because the sensations you pick up through them transmit instant impressions. You learn to assess through touch where to work on the body beneath your hands. The wonder and joy created through this form of expression is simple yet profound. Each time you find an area that needs a specific touch the excitement of discovery is breathtaking.

What Is Touch?

The first sense to be used in life is that of touch. Babies are cuddled, hugged, nursed, and wrapped in welcome upon entry into the world. For infants, touch not only signals safety, it triggers the growth hormone, giving the go-ahead to grow. For children of all ages, normal metabolism depends on touch. Families live together in close quarters, sharing space, touching each other, and reassuring children and adults, alike, that they are safe and all is well. We need to be touched to survive.

Touch not only encourages growth, it is an essential ingredient in the development of a well-adjusted being. Loving touch promotes spiritual, physical, mental, and emotional well-being. To be a happy, loving, intelligent, stable baby, child, and finally adult, constant tender caring touch is necessary. Babies begin touching while still carried inside their mother. Upon entering the world the first sense a baby demonstrates is the need to touch, whether by rooting about to nurse or grasping with little hands to feel mother. There is no conscious thought involved, rather the driving instinct that allows the newborn to respond to the sense of touch.

Touch Is a Sense

The sensation of touch occurs because of receptors in the skin. Receptors are sense organs that receive information, known as stimulus, from outside or inside the body and then transmit this information as a nerve impulse to the brain, where it becomes feeling. Although thought is not involved, the brain identifies the sensation, bringing our awareness to the feeling.

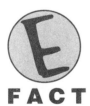

FACT

Touch, or tactile sensation, is connected to receptors known as mechanoreceptors, which are capable of picking up three kinds (or levels) of sensations: touch, pressure, and vibration.

The receptors that lie just below the top layer of skin respond to stimulation that results in the sensation of touch. These touch receptors give you the ability to notice touch whether it is light or discriminatory. When experiencing a light touch, you recognize that something has touched the skin but you may not recognize exactly what is touching or where. Feather-light touch skimming the surface of the skin creates a tingling sensation that remains even after the fingers have moved on. With a discriminatory touch, you know precisely where your body is being touched as the firm pressure of fingers and hands keeps you grounded in the moment. The touch receptors for pressure and vibration are found deeper in the body in the lower levels of tissue. These sensations of pressure and vibration generally cover a broader area of the body and last longer than do the lighter or discriminatory touch sensations.

Temperature and Pain Receptors

The response to hot and cold is known as thermoreceptive sensation. Thermoreceptive receptors are free nerve endings that respond to environmental temperatures, both internal and external. These receptors are found in the skin, the tissue, and the organs.

Pain receptors, known as nociceptors, are free nerve endings that are found most everywhere in the body, and are essential for survival. Pain is the reaction to overstimulation of the touch and temperature sensations. As these nociceptors respond to stimuli they alert the body to danger, letting you know that something is wrong.

Introducing Touch to Others and Ourselves

Your skin can sense different levels of touch. You can recognize the light whisper of a soft breeze as well as the harsh pounding of ocean surf against your skin. You also have the ability to adapt to touch, such as when you feel the continued weight of your winter coat for a minute or two and then no longer recognize the added burden. The touch receptors in your skin become adjusted to the constant presence of the coat and allow your awareness to shift elsewhere.

Touch as Communication

Touch is a form of communication. You gently touch your baby, rubbing her back, reminding her that you are here keeping her safe. You embrace your partner, then stay in close contact, letting your body brush slightly against his, keeping the connection. You greet a friend with a bear hug. You hold both hands in warm welcome as you connect with an honored peer or mentor. You may lightly touch the person you are speaking to, as a way of staying connected or punctuating the points of discussion. You meet someone for the first time, and you shake hands, briefly yet firmly.

Through each of these encounters touch is the medium of communication. So much is said through touch, especially in massage where you communicate through different levels. The touch may be firm, or deep. At times the touch may be so light as to convey the heat of energy without actually touching.

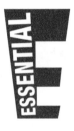

Always gear the massage to the need of the receiver at that particular time. Find out if there are any painful or injured areas. Ask if the receiver is anxious, under a great deal of stress, or has any other emotional issues. Is the massage at the end of the day for relaxation or is the receiver returning to work and needs an energizing break?

Always talk with your massage partner first, recognizing areas of sensitivity as well as creating a comfort zone. Once you have prepared the person who is receiving, the different strokes will become the "words" used during the session. You and those you work on will enjoy tenfold the journey of massage as you set an intention to always use appropriate touch.

Intuition and Touch

Intuition is that part of you that lets you know where to work and what to do without any cues from the receiver. You may get an actual feeling or you may have a thought or even a picture in your mind of what will feel good to the recipient. Always listen to your intuitive self and be guided by what you feel. Touch through intuition adds depth to your massage, allowing you to be more than a technician.

Touching someone will often trigger a response in your own body. You may be massaging someone and feel a slight twinge of pain in your left shoulder. Massage the same shoulder on your receiver using your body as a guide, gauging what strokes and pressure to use. Trust what you are feeling and you will find as you work that the pain in your shoulder or wherever will dissipate.

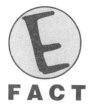

FACT

On September 9, 1971 the Exploratorium in the Palace of Fine Arts in San Francisco opened a permanent exhibit called the Tactile Dome. Housed in a geodesic dome in total darkness, the exhibit provides an hour and fifteen minutes of finding one's way through a darkened maze, sensing only by touch. The dark path is an experience depending solely on the ability of the participants to walk, crawl, and feel their way through many different materials.

Touching with Compassion

Loving and compassionate touch creates an atmosphere conducive to self-healing. Caring about the well-being of the person you are working on allows you to give the best massage ever. Always enter into the giving space with the intention to allow whatever is appropriate for the person receiving.

Giving Security Through Touch

Wholeness of body, mind, and spirit is a concept you will be encouraging in all those you work with. Through touch you allow a loving healing to take place. Your caring message can be conveyed to the receiver through touch. Kind touch says, "You are now in a safe place; you may release all tension and relax, totally."

The touch of massage lets the recipient know now is the time to clear and cleanse, to let go of the toxins the body holds. The body welcomes release and is thankful for the compassion transmitted through the gentle touch of the giver. Muscles hold tension, which is the result of our reaction to stress, and massage is a key used to unlock this impairment. Often folks push unresolved issues into the body, rather than deal with them.

Holding emotions in the body will cause that part of the body to eventually freeze, essentially restricting the function of that piece, whether it is a muscle, organ, or bone. As we lose contact with a part of the body, we generally reject that area, attracting overall dysfunction. The muscle will become tight, the bone may ache, and the organ does not realize its full capacity. Kind touch recognizes the need to celebrate the entire body and embrace every piece.

You can help the receiver learn to rejoice in his or her body, to accept it as it is, rather than how he or she would like it to be. Often the part of the body that is ignored or rejected will not function in the way the operator desires. The massage therapist teaches the receiver how to experience the body as whole, even with its restrictions. Compassionate touch listens to the body, working to allow relaxation by teaching the receiver to rejoice in the wholeness of the body.

Teaching Self-Love

Massage done with compassion creates an environment that encourages connection to self and approval of self. Self-criticism is held in the body as tension, resulting in painful muscles, achy bones, and congestion in the organs. Self-love releases the blocks that screen out the balance necessary for wholeness. Understanding that distress indicates imbalance allows the receiver to begin the path to wellness.

Some conditions held in the body are chronic, meaning they are long-term life conditions. Through compassion and love, massage can help folks who have such chronic health conditions learn to accept but not disregard them. You can help people to look at themselves as living with their condition, but not being limited by it. Embracing the concept of whole wellness allows people to choose holistic healing modalities, such as massage, that will help them live with chronic conditions yet not be ruled by them.

You can assist your receiver along his or her journey in healing. The compassionate touch you use helps the receiver to become focused on his or her body in love and welcome recognition. Kind touch says, "I am worthy of love and I love my body the way it is." You can support the concept of self-love and appreciation by teaching the recipient to acknowledge the gift of life. The more a person accepts the body she lives in the more the body will change. As a person grows to love her body, the person will work harder to honor its well-being.

Appropriate Touch

Massage is all about the right touch. It is important to know when to use a certain stroke in massage, how much pressure to apply, and how long to stay in one area. It is equally as important to know when to work on an area and when not to. Always check with your receiver before massaging to understand where the massage should be focused.

A feeling of well-being and inner calmness is the result of a healing massage. The contract between the giver and receiver recognizes the need of the receiver to feel completely at ease, confident in the ability of the giver to appropriately provide what is needed. You offer compassionate touch together with respect and limit setting. The boundaries established in this sacred contract are workable and appropriate.

When Touch Is Inappropriate

Massage is a wonderful healing tool for relaxation and relief from muscle tension. Massage helps people to release stress and to feel stronger, healthier, and happier. Circulation is improved with massage, giving the skin a refreshed appearance. There are times, however, when massage is not indicated, and there are areas of the body that are either too sensitive for massage or are inappropriate to touch. Use your common sense whenever you prepare to massage someone.

Medical Conditions

There will be times when underlying conditions indicate that massage is not advisable at the time. If the receiver has a temperature higher than normal from a fever or an infection, massage is not the best form of relaxation at that time. High temperature is the body's way of fighting off germs that are attacking the immune system; therefore, the receiver's fever indicates that his or her body is working to find the invaders and eliminate them. Massage would interfere with the natural process of the body so it is better to wait until the temperature is back to normal.

Massage is not a good idea if someone is in a lot of pain, even if you know the pain is due to a muscle spasm. When muscles are actively involved in an intense spasm, which is greater than a muscle cramp, massage is not helpful. If someone has such a powerful spasm that movement is close to impossible, please suggest that person go to a professional massage therapist. Sometimes even a professional will not work on the spasm and will make a referral to a medical practitioner.

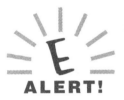

Pain is the body's way of letting you know there is a serious problem and may be the signal of an internal difficulty. Always point this out to your receiver and encourage him or her to immediately see a doctor. Do not give a massage until a medical professional has been consulted.

Someone who has difficulty breathing should not be massaged. A person feeling disoriented, anxious, or panicky is not a candidate for massage, either. And finally, elderly folks suffering with osteoporosis need the permission of their doctor before you give a massage—very gently.

Areas of Sensitivity

Some areas of the body are best massaged with a feather touch or not at all. The space in the center of the throat is an area you can stay away from because it is very sensitive. The neck area in general must be massaged gently, because nerves and arteries are close to the surface and very sensitive, too. The face also has sections that should not be touched: Do not massage the eyes, or even around the soft eye area; and it is best to touch the ears very gently, staying away from the spot just under and behind the bottom of the ear.

The arms have a few areas that you should touch softly. The armpit is very sensitive and often ticklish, so you may not be able to massage there. The inside upper arm, which is filled with nerves, should be massaged gently from the armpit down to the elbow. The elbow holds the "funny bone," a region that you know can cause a lot of pain if touched too hard. Not funny!

The legs have a few parts that are sensitive, too. The inside of the top of the leg, where it connects to your pelvis is very sensitive, so do not press there because you can cut off the circulation, and it hurts, too. The back of the knee must be massaged very gently with a feather touch, and the back of the heel is also filled with nerves, so go softly there, too.

The stomach is an especially touchy place—touch too gently and it feels ticklish; use too much pressure and it is painful. Massage very steadily yet gently and that should be just right. Some people may not like to be pushed and prodded in the stomach area, and that's okay; just move on. The lower back above and below the waistline is where the kidneys are found, and is a place you should massage gently. Lastly, the spine itself is not to be worked on; you can massage on either side but do not press on the spine.

Hostile Touch

Never ever work on someone if you are angry with that person. Wait until you have discussed the issue that caused the feeling before you engage in any touch therapy. Because massage is a wonderful relaxant and instills a feeling of pleasure if done appropriately, touch should always convey the intent of unconditional giving, never anger.

If you are involved in a power struggle or conflict of any kind with the receiver, resolve the affair before you give the massage. Even anger not directed at your receiver may be felt, so wait until you feel better before actually giving a massage. Remember that massage is a physical and an energetic therapy, and what you feel will be transmitted through touch.

Genital Areas

Massage should never create a feeling of anxiety in the person receiving. Always make your recipient feel safe. Make sure to drape areas that are not being worked on, especially the genital parts of the body. Leave no doubt in the recipient's mind that you are going to work appropriately. Through your confident touch and your no-nonsense manner the receiver will always feel safe and secure.

Light Touch

Whether you are giving or receiving, the quality of the touch is key to the enjoyment of the massage. Initially, contact should be light yet constant as an introduction into the energetic space of another person. You can place your hands lightly on the receiver's back, and this establishes a strong connection. Touching lightly yet firmly establishes the foundation for the healing environment.

The Effects of Light Touch

A smooth light touch stirs memories from early childhood. Using light touch to design the safe environment of massage, you remind the receiver of soft blankets and loving arms. The recipient will sink down and relax, releasing the initial layer of tension as your light touch gives permission to let go.

Relax your breathing so you can tune in to the breathing rhythm of the person on the table. See if the breathing pattern of the receiver is smooth and calm or irregular and restricted. The rhythm of the breath lets you know how tense or relaxed your recipient is. Your soft touch is the signal to unwind, to let go of all troubles, to be still and calm.

Using Light Touch

The quality of your massage is expressed through your ability to provide consistent, easy touch. Place your hands lightly on the receiver to begin receiving information about the body you are going to work on. Use your hands and fingers to find areas of tension as you move easily across the receiving body, gently stroking the body with soft, calming movements. Tension is recognized as tightness in the muscle, which makes the skin feel hard under your fingers. A shift in temperature from one part of the body to another will denote tension as well. Practice maintaining contact as you gently move your hands over the skin and muscles, assessing areas that are taut and even areas that may be too relaxed.

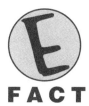

FACT

A muscle that feels loose and flat means the normal tone that creates the round firm shape of a healthy muscle is not present. An area that is too relaxed may signal the beginning of atrophy due to lack of use. Massage is an important tool in assisting muscle exercise.

Deep Pressure

Light touch evolves into deep pressure as you move into the troubled areas of the body. Your hands act as your eyes, sensing where to work lightly and where to progress deeply, as your hands communicate to the body and the body communicates to you. Using deep pressure ensures steady, sustained contact, touching to the core of the distress.

Applying Deep Pressure

Your hands and fingers are alert to finding areas that need deeper pressure, identifying knotted areas of tension. Shoulders and back muscles often require a deeper touch, once you have warmed up the body with light touch, which opens the regions that need deeper work. As you move into these areas feel the tightness under the skin. Slow steady movement allows you to deepen the touch, effectively working the knots out.

Deep pressure is used to release inflammation and to break up scar tissue. Scar tissue adversely affects the function of the area it is connected to, often forming adhesions. Deep massage helps to break up these adhesions as well.

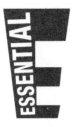

ESSENTIAL

Adhesions are the result of tissues joining abnormally. They are found around areas of inflammation as a result of tissue damage often caused by surgery, after which they form along the site of an incision. Adhesions may need to be removed; this can be done surgically or through deep massage.

Move Your Body

The best way to apply deep pressure is to move your body. Try this exercise. Put on your favorite reggae, hip-hop, or rock music and get ready to boogie! Have someone lie on the table and place your hands on his or her upper back, with your body at the head of the table. Have your feet planted firmly on the ground, about a shoulder's width apart. Let your hands rest gently on the back and move side to side in time with the music; remember to bend your knees.

Notice how your hands begin to press into the back without any effort from you. Place one leg behind you, moving into a yoga-like warrior stance. Your hands will shift slightly; one may be a bit higher than the other. Keep moving in time with the music, and your hands will automatically press in deeper and deeper as you move rhythmically with the music.

Begin slow circular motions with your hands, as you continue to move. As you move toward the table your fingertips press in deeply. As you move away from the table the heels of your palms apply the greater pressure.

Practice this type of moving on different parts of the receiver's body. Feel the rhythm rather than think about the movements. You are finding the groove that works for you, setting the memory of movement into your massage. Your body rhythm is far more effective than plain pressing with your hands. By using your entire body, the receiver feels deep pressure that is steady and assured. By employing your entire body, not just your hands and arms, you ensure that you can continue to massage for many years as no part of your body is overworked.

The world of massage is a safe, comfortable place. Enjoy the feeling of giving as you receive. When you give a massage you are also getting.

The pure joy of giving peace and comfort to another creates a sensation of peace and comfort in the giver as well. The magnificent world of touch awaits you.

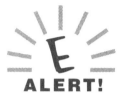

ALERT!

Moving your body rhythmically allows you to apply deep pressure without pain to the receiver or you, the giver. Massage may generate a small amount of discomfort, what is termed "good pain," in the receiver. However, excessive pressure causing real discomfort will cause the muscles to tense up, creating injury. Remember to move, move, move!

Chapter 3

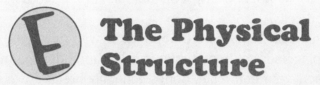

The Physical Structure

The human body is a fabulous self-contained unit that functions in a state of perfect balance—most of the time. The various structures that make up the body communicate in a number of ways to keep the functions operating properly. The different structural levels ultimately group together into body systems that work together cooperatively; one system cannot operate without the combined efforts of every other system in the body.

The Skeletal System

The skeletal system helps us move and protects our organs. It is composed of cartilage and bones that connect to and support the body. The skeleton contains 206 bones that are attached to the body by ligaments, tendons, and muscles. Bones work in conjunction with other parts of the body to keep us healthy. For example, bones store minerals and produce blood cells.

Your body continually replaces old bone tissue with new bone tissue. This perpetual replacement of bone tissue is called remodeling, and it continues throughout your entire life. Bones generally break down old bone in the center and form new bone from the outside. Along with the process of removal and replacement, remodeling places bones in the position of serving as the calcium storage unit for the body.

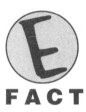

FACT

Calcium is necessary for many functions. For example, muscles need calcium to perform the operation of contraction; nerve cells require calcium to perform the job of conduction; and bones need calcium to remain strong. Calcium is supplied to all the tissues of the body through the blood. The body constantly recycles the supply of calcium throughout the organs.

Makeup of the Muscles

To actually move the body, the framework of the skeleton works through contraction and relaxation of muscles. Your body is 50 percent muscle! Muscles make the body warm, keep the body stable, and see to it that your internal organs operate. There are more than 600 skeletal muscles in the body, all of which can benefit from massage, either directly or indirectly.

Types of Muscles

Muscle tissue is divided into three types: skeletal, cardiac, and smooth. Skeletal muscles are also known as voluntary muscles because they move at your command. Skeletal muscles form the shape of the body and move the skeletal bones they are attached to.

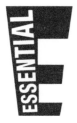

To walk, skip, run, or jump, you move your muscles at will. You can catch and throw something, type on a computer, turn pages of a book, drive a car, and dance all night because your skeletal muscles move voluntarily. Chewing food, smiling, talking, singing, or frowning are all voluntary movements performed by you.

The heart muscle is known as the cardiac muscle. Cardiac muscle tissue is found only in the heart and provides the movement necessary for the heart to beat. This muscle is an involuntary muscle, meaning you have no control over whether or not your heart will beat. Cardiac muscle must be fed a constant supply of oxygen to support it while the muscle contracts and relaxes at an average rate of 75 times a minute.

Smooth muscle is also an involuntary muscle, but this one is found inside organs, blood vessels, and at the point in the skin where hair follicles are attached. Smooth muscle tissue can stretch to a great length without loosing its elasticity. When the bladder or stomach is full, this muscle is able to stretch to accommodate the fullness. When the stomach or bladder is empty, the muscles return to their normal size, ready to be filled again.

The makeup of muscle fiber dictates whether or not it can regenerate. Some skeletal muscles have the ability to renew themselves, and smooth muscles can regenerate considerably, but cardiac muscles cannot. Exercise increases the flow of blood and oxygen, which contributes to the growth and renewal of skeletal muscles.

Functions of the Muscles

Muscles perform motion, maintain posture, and produce heat. They do this work through contractions that occur when an internal chemical process turns energy into movement. Some muscle motion is observable, such as running, dancing, talking, singing, and typing. Other motion you can't see but takes place when you digest your food, when your heart beats, or when you eliminate waste. Your muscles sustain your posture by keeping you sitting or standing without falling over. Lastly, the contraction of muscles produces and maintains body heat. Think about how warm you get when you exercise; this is a perfect example of muscles at work.

Massage and Skeletal Muscle Tissue

Skeletal muscle is the type of muscle primarily affected by massage. This muscle consists of connective tissue, blood, and lymph, as well as nerve tissue. Blood and lymph supply food to the muscles and take away the waste. Nerves send the impulses for movement and sensation. Connective tissue makes up the bulk of the muscle.

Massage works on the connective layers of muscle tissue, and makes the muscles feel good. Systematic and steady massaging of muscles releases toxins that may be causing fatigue. Massage also helps to improve muscle tone and prevent muscle spasms.

The Nervous System

The nervous system is one of the systems responsible for homeostasis; that is, keeping the body in balance. The nervous system responds to changes in the body through nerve impulses, adjusting body functions as needed. Homeostasis and whole health depend upon the proper operation of the nervous system, in cooperative partnership with the endocrine system.

The three main functions of the nervous system are to sense, respond, and integrate. The sensory part of the nervous system monitors the stimuli that cause environmental changes inside and outside your body, by checking with all your senses. The response part monitors stimuli to your muscles or your glands. The integrative part analyzes the information received from the senses and assists in directing the motor response.

The nervous system is divided into two sections, the central nervous system (CNS) and the peripheral nervous system (PNS). The brain and the spinal cord make up the CNS while the PNS is composed of the cranial and spinal nerves. The CNS interprets sensory information sending out signals to muscles and glands as well as creating thoughts and emotions and storing memories. The PNS is responsible for sensory and motor impulses throughout the entire body generating voluntary and involuntary responses.

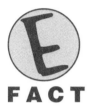

FACT

The PNS uses the sensory nerves to send messages to the brain, and the motor nerves to conduct the messages from the brain out to the rest of the body. The skin is a main transmitter of both kinds of messages, receiving and giving information. As a result, massage is a valuable tool in stimulating or relaxing the nervous system.

Massage and the Nervous System

Massage affects the nerves, which in turn contributes to stimulation of most of the body functions. As the muscles and connective tissue relax, the nerves feeding all areas of the body seem to perform more efficiently. As the nervous system functions at a higher level the body responds more effectively, reaching its highest potential. Good health is maintained through regular massage.

The Endocrine System

The endocrine system works in rhythm with the nervous system. The nervous system sends electrical messages to direct the body, while the endocrine system sends chemical messages. Endocrine glands secrete hormones into the bloodstream to keep the body in balance. Hormones from these glands are involved in your growth and development and are key to your reproductive process. Hormones are responsible for the production and nourishment of newborns, and also help the body deal with demands such as infection or stress.

Endocrine glands and organs containing endocrine tissues include the following:

- **Pituitary gland:** Secretes many hormones including those that control reproductive functions.
- **Pineal gland:** Produces the hormone that influences sleep patterns.
- **Thyroid gland:** Regulates metabolism, growth, and development, and the nervous system.
- **Parathyroid glands:** Help regulate the levels of calcium and other elements in the blood.
- **Thymus gland:** Helps produce cells that fight infection.
- **Suprarenal (adrenal) glands:** Secrete many hormones, including those that help the body deal with stress.
- **Pancreas:** Produces hormones that regulate blood sugar and help with digestion.
- **Ovaries:** Produce female sex hormones.
- **Testes:** Produce male sex hormones.

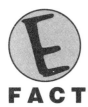

FACT

The other type of gland in the body is the exocrine gland. Exocrine glands have ducts that transport the products of these glands into the body or onto the surface of the body. The exocrine glands are sweat glands, tear ducts, oil glands, digestive glands, and mucus glands.

The Working of the Heart and Blood

The heart, blood, and blood vessels are all part of the system known as the cardiovascular or circulatory system. The heart is a muscle that works constantly, 24 hours a day, beating 60 to 80 times a minute, pumping all the blood in your body through one full cycle, once every minute! Blood circulates through your body carrying oxygen and nutrients through a system of blood vessels. A healthy heart can grow even stronger and healthier through exercise.

Blood Circulation

The heart has four chambers known as the right and left atrium and the right and left ventricle. Blood travels through the body's veins and enters the right atrium. From there it is pumped into the right ventricle, and then into the lungs for oxygenation and removal of carbon dioxide and other wastes. The oxygenated blood then returns to the left atrium and passes down into the left ventricle. The left ventricle pumps the blood out to the rest of the body through arteries where it eventually reaches tiny branches called capillaries. From there the deoxygenated blood makes a return cycle through the veins and back to the heart. Valves in the heart stop the blood from flowing the wrong way.

Blood Pressure

Blood pressure is what forces the nutrients and oxygen into the cells of the body, which is why balanced blood pressure is important to good health. By maintaining a good level of pressure the body keeps the blood vessels and heart healthy. Exercise, nutrition, and reduction of stress are all holistic ways to keep the heart functioning at its best. Massage is very effective in supporting the circulatory system, because it encourages the removal of waste and keeps oxygen moving through the body.

The Lymphatic System

The lymphatic system and the circulatory system work together. The lymphatic system consists of lymph, lymph nodes, lymph vessels, and lymphatic ducts. Lymph is a straw-colored fluid that is transported by blood vessels to fight infectious invasion to the body. The lymph nodes contain lymphocytes that help to remove bacteria from the lymphatic fluid before it reaches the blood. The lymph combined with the other organs of the immune system (thymus, spleen, and tonsils) hold the position of first guard in the body. Everything in this system flows toward the heart, continuously picking up waste along the way. Massage helps to keep the lymph system healthy, contributing to the body's ability to release toxins.

The Respiratory System

The upper respiratory system consists of the nose and the pharynx. Air enters through the nose where it is warmed, moistened, and filtered. Hair in the nose filters out larger dust particles, while mucus traps the remaining dust. Small structures called cilia move the mucus and dust into the pharynx, which is the throat. From the pharynx the mucus is either expelled or swallowed.

The lower respiratory system is made up of the larynx, trachea, bronchi, and lungs. The larynx is the structure that contains the vocal cords, and is sometimes referred to as the voice box. The larynx allows air to pass to the trachea, or windpipe. The trachea flows into two structures, the right and left bronchi, which are air ducts that transport air to and from the lungs. The oxygen from the air in the lungs passes into the blood and flows through the body bringing nourishment to the cells. The waste matter in the form of carbon dioxide is moved out of the cells, into the blood, back into the lungs, and out of the body. Oxygen remains in the body and the carbon dioxide is gone. The exchange of gases is complete.

The Digestive System

Food supplies nutrients that build and repair body tissues, and provides energy. The ability to nourish cells is realized through the chemical conversion of solid food to a usable form through the process of digestion. The digestive system comprises the organs that break down food into usable units: the pharynx (the throat), the esophagus (connects the throat to the stomach), the stomach, and the small and large intestines.

The digestive system also contains accessory organs that produce enzymes needed to digest food. The liver produces bile, a necessary tool to break down fat in the body. The gallbladder stores bile until it is needed. The pancreas, a digestive gland that secretes enzymes to break down proteins, carbohydrates, and fats, sends these chemicals into the small intestine to assist the work of the stomach.

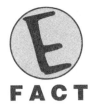

FACT

The liver has more than 500 functions. It is the largest gland in the body, producing bile to break down fat, storing important vitamins and minerals, as well as producing amino acids. The liver is the detoxifying gland, cleaning the body of such substances as drugs, alcohol, nicotine, and other toxic chemicals.

The digestive system works to ingest, move, digest, absorb, and eliminate food. Ingestion of food is the process of eating. Movement of the food along the gastrointestinal tract occurs through a series of muscular contractions. Digestion of food involves chewing as well as the churning and mixing done in the intestines; once the mechanical process is complete food continues to be digested through the addition of chemical enzymes. Absorption of food occurs when the nutrients of digested food are moved into cells throughout your body via the blood and lymph. Elimination occurs through excretion of the indigestible matter from the body.

Elimination of Waste

True elimination of waste involves many of the body's systems. The respiratory system releases carbon dioxide from the body, a major waste product from the cells. The skin allows waste to leave as you sweat. The digestive system removes waste through excretion. The urinary system keeps the body in homeostasis by removing waste and replenishing the blood.

The kidneys along with the ureters, the bladder, and the urethra comprise the urinary system. The kidneys are responsible for the production of urine, and the other organs either store or remove it. The kidneys also filter the blood, allowing nutrients in and keeping wastes out. All of the body's blood is cleaned and filtered by the kidneys every day. These two small organs also keep the balance of water, salt, and potassium in the body. This function keeps you from retaining excess fluid, which can cause swelling in your hands, feet, legs, and other parts of your body.

The ureters are responsible for carrying urine away from the kidneys to the bladder, where urine is stored. Once the bladder is full, the pressure of the volume allows the bladder to release the stored urine through the urethra, a tiny tube traveling from the bladder to the outside of the body.

The Integumentary System

The integumentary system is composed of different but related tissue groups that combine to form an organ system that covers and protects the body. This system is composed of skin, hair, nails, sweat and oil glands, and nerve endings, but in massage, our primary focus is on the skin. Skin is our contact with the physical world, the vehicle for sensations of touching and being touched. Skin protects the body—it is the body's first defense. We even reflect our emotions through our skin, either by color, expression, or temperature. Massage is a way to keep the skin healthy, supple, and strong.

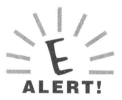

ALERT!

All skin benefits as ultraviolet rays from the sun increase the growth of melanin, producing a tan, protecting the skin from damaging radiation. Of course, too much exposure to UV rays can lead to skin cancer. Moderate exposure to the sun and the use of sunscreen will ensure proper melanin production without the damaging effects.

The Three Layers of Skin

The top layer of skin, the epidermis, is made up of five separate layers, which are responsible for things like protecting the skin and monitoring the passage of water. The epidermis also contains nerve endings for touch. The epithelial tissue that makes up the top layer of skin is continuously regenerating, reproducing cells that push up to the surface. As the cells move up through the layers they begin to die, eventually reaching the top layer of our skin, which then sheds the dead cells, and the renewal process continues. The rejuvenation of skin takes about three to six weeks.

The cells responsible for pigmentation of the skin are also found in the epidermis. As new cells sprout from the basal layer, some of these cells develop melanin granules. Cells called melanocytes produce the melanin that is responsible for the color of the skin. Everyone is born with the same number of melanocytes; it is the amount of melanin produced that determines skin color. Dark skin produces more melanin than light skin, giving extra protection from aging and environmental damage.

The second layer of skin, the dermis, is the layer that sits under and is connected to the epidermis. Blood vessels and additional nerve endings are found here, as well as the fibers that give skin its extensibility and elasticity. The dermis also contains hair follicles as well as sweat and oil glands.

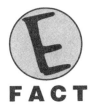

FACT

Extensibility is the capacity of the skin to stretch, such as during pregnancy, weight gain, or excessive swelling. Elasticity enables the skin to return to its original shape. At times the skin may stretch too much, causing tiny tears in the dermis that show up as stretch marks.

The third and deepest layer of the skin is the subcutaneous layer. This layer is made up of adipose tissue, which is fat, a necessary element to healthy skin. This layer of tissue connects the dermis to the bone and muscle beneath. The subcutaneous layer provides shape to the body and provides an extra cushion of protection for the skin above.

What Skin Does

The function of skin, actually of the entire integumentary system, is extensive. The skin is an efficient regulatory system essential to the maintenance of the entire body. It provides protection, produces vitamins, maintains and regulates body temperature, and removes toxic waste. A protein called keratin creates a waterproof shield along the surface of the skin, protecting the body from fluid loss and fluid gain. The skin serves as a line of defense against microorganisms and environmental invaders, such as bacteria, viruses, chemicals, and radiation. It also acts as the first barricade against physical injury. The skin is our largest sensory organ.

Types of Skin

Skin has many colors and textures due to many factors. Genetic makeup dictates some of the conditions of our skin. So do sun exposure, what we eat, whether or not we smoke, and other environmental factors.

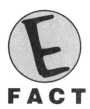

FACT

Wrinkles are evidence of early unprotected moments in the sun although they show up on the skin in later years. Research has proven that people who stay out of the sun look six to ten years younger than folks who are constantly sun exposed. Without a lifetime of sun exposure, our skin could remain supple and young-looking until our seventies.

We have all seen ads that talk about different types of skin—too dry, too oily, or just right, whatever that might be! Actually skin is an individual characteristic owned solely by you. Your skin is affected by your internal conditions such as hormone fluctuations, and by external conditions where you live such as weather or sun exposure. Makeup, skin creams, skin cleansers—any type of skin care product—also put demands on your skin. There are three main types of skin:

- **Oily skin** comes from an overproduction of sebum, which normally allows skin to be soft, smooth, and pliable. Blackheads are formed when pores are clogged by too much sebum.
- **Dry skin** is often caused by environment and age. Dry climate or winter air pulls much of the moisture out of our skin, leaving it taut and dry. With age comes dry skin, because the top layer of the epidermis is less able to hold water in.
- **Sensitive skin** can be the result of allergies, overexposure to chemicals, or too much sun. Cosmetics contain chemicals and fragrances that may cause sensitivity in some people. Most folks have sensitive skin at some time in their lives.

The Effects of Massage on the Skin

The skin receives tremendous benefit from massage. Massage helps to remove the top layer of dead cells, improving the condition of the skin and making it look and feel healthier. Circulation is improved, bringing a new supply of blood to the sebaceous glands. As the fresh blood circulates, the sebaceous glands produce more sebum to keep the skin soft and supple. Improved circulation also stimulates the sweat glands, allowing for the release of toxins. At the same time, the blood vessels expand, providing nutrients to the skin. Massage helps to release fatty tissue from the body as well as break up scar tissue.

Massage is essential to the support and function of the body systems. As massage reduces the stress in the body it allows the body and its various systems to function at the highest level possible. Massage is a preventive tool as well as a remedial benefit. Whether you have great health or are suffering from a chronic issue, massage is an important and helpful adjunct to better health.

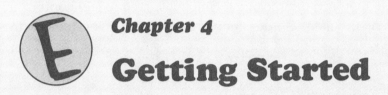

Chapter 4

Getting Started

Massage can be as fancy or as simple as you make it. Giving a massage is pleasurable and can be done anywhere; it takes only two people—a giver and a receiver. Whether you are outside or in, at home or at work, have a free afternoon or a quick lunch break, performing and receiving massage is nearly always a possibility. The important point is to relax and enjoy. Receiving a massage or giving one can be a terrific experience!

Preparing Yourself

Massage is a hands-on technique. When you think about touching someone it is good practice to allow yourself to relax and de-stress before actually beginning the massage. Remember, touch is a vehicle of communication; therefore it is important to have calm, loving intention when you approach the recipient. Helping someone feel good is always a joyful event; the natural process of massage is an enjoyable way to spread the love.

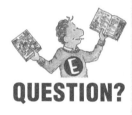

QUESTION?

How do I create this calm, loving intention?
There are many ways to generate and maintain a relaxed, caring attitude. You can meditate or exercise before working. Or you can give yourself a massage while listening to your favorite music. A guided visualization is also a constructive tool. Communing with nature is helpful, too.

As you become familiar with various styles of relaxation you will find those that fit you. Some of the best forms of relaxation teach us how to listen to our own body, and when we understand what we need we can become aware of the needs of others. A large part of massage work is tuning in to the person you are working on. If your massage partner has indicated that her neck hurts, that is the area you will work on. You can bet when you place your hands on her shoulders they will feel tight, too. Remember to relax and be calm as you approach the receiver, and your hands will become your eyes, helping you to discover what areas are in need.

To relax your body, stand tall with your shoulders relaxed and feet shoulder-width apart, with your arms hanging loosely at your sides. Close your eyes and inhale deeply bringing your shoulders up to your ears. Exhale and push your shoulders down feeling your neck stretch up. Repeat this three times.

Continue the relaxed stance and let your head fall gently to the right, remembering to breathe. On the inhalation bring your head up and gently drop it to the left as you exhale. Repeat this once more to the right and the left, then return to the original position with your head upright. Clasp your hands behind your back and step your right foot and leg out in front to a slightly bent knee posture. Stretch your arms away from your back, feeling the muscles release. Bring your arms down, hands still clasped behind, and your right leg back in. Step your left leg out and while bent at the knee stretch your arms out in the back, hands still together.

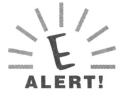

ALERT!

It is essential to know that you cannot "fix" anyone. Rather, you assist or facilitate healing as your inner body wisdom carries on its work. Massage is a wonderful tool to help us feel better, but if someone has unidentified pain you must send that person to a health-care professional.

Lastly start by standing tall, reaching your arms up to the sky, joining your hands together above your head. Spread your legs slightly wider than shoulder-width apart and gently bend forward, scooping your belly in while reaching down with your hands. Stretch only as far as comfortable, bending your knees slightly. Come back up slowly to easy standing position. You are ready to begin.

Consider the Receiver

Before you actually work on your massage partner spend a few minutes discussing his or her needs. Listen to the issues that concern the receiver. Every massage is relaxing, although some address specific problems. Massage is used to help an ache feel better, or relieve a stiff muscle, or relax the whole body. What exactly is the receiver looking for?

Establish a routine with yourself that allows time to address the needs and concerns of the recipient before you actually begin the massage. Every person is an individual with requirements that are particular to his or her body. There are many different ways to proceed with a massage routine. The idea is to remain flexible and give a relaxing, effective massage.

Be Aware of Your Receiver's Needs

Remember that when deciding how to give each massage you will be relying not only on what the individual is requesting but also on your own observations. Always check for restrictions in mobility and be aware of any chronic conditions that might prohibit a normal massage.

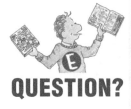

QUESTION?

What is a chronic condition?
Any long-term disease, such as diabetes or arthritis, is considered to be chronic because it is long-term or nonending. High blood pressure or thyroid disease represent other examples of long-term or chronic conditions. Something that will heal, like a broken leg or a poison ivy rash, is an acute condition.

Age plays a factor in the choices you will have when administrating a massage. What the receiver will be doing following the massage is another important piece of information. Find out if there are any previous or present injuries or surgeries; this will dictate your pressure and style.

Consider the time available also. What are you able to accomplish in the time you both have allowed for this activity? Giving someone a massage late at night when you are tired is not such a great idea. A massage at lunch is fine, if you both have allowed enough time for what is needed. Beginning a massage just before the kids come home for supper is not the best use of time. Plan to give massages when both you and the receiver have enough quiet time and space.

Get Comfortable

Once you have determined that you and your receiver are ready, make him as comfortable as possible. Use bolsters, wedges, and pillows—even rolled towels—to provide extra comfort. Make sure you have enough sheets and blankets to cover the receiver, making him feel safe and secure.

It is also your responsibility to provide a quiet, private, clean environment for the massage. Prepare to devote this time to your receiver—turn off the phone! Whether you have an entire healing space or a beautiful screened area, the atmosphere must feel comfortable and protected for your recipient and for you. Take the time to create a warm, loving, secure space that is inviting as well as sheltered. The rule of thumb when preparing for a massage is to make sure you and your space are neat and clean. Keep the space clear of clutter and free of dust. Set the tone with lighting and music, forming a space that is inviting and restful.

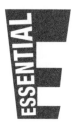

Palpation is an integral part of massage. Palpating means to touch the muscle tissue in order to gather information. You feel with your touch what your eyes do not see. You can see a swollen area, but your fingers will tell you if the area is hard and hot or soft and filled with fluid.

When Massage Is Called For

Massage is a useful tool in many ways for many situations. You can use massage to promote relaxation. You can use massage to reduce pain, to encourage healing, and to dispel scar tissue and adhesions. You can also use massage to help restore mobility, improve circulation, and aid in digestion and elimination.

Relaxing Stiff Muscles

Massage can ease stiff muscles and muscle spasms caused by physical stress. In relaxing tense muscles, massage can also ease mental and emotional stress, a benefit often recognized by people seeking relief with massage. Receiving massage helps the receiver make some positive changes in body, mind, and spirit.

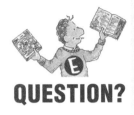

QUESTION?

What is a muscle spasm?
Properly functioning muscles are smooth with no discernable kinks. A spasm causes a kind of bump to appear along the muscle line, like a kink or knot in a rope. Stress on a muscle may cause these twists and kinks to appear, interfering with proper muscle operation.

Stress and repetitive motion are often the cause of tight, stiff muscles. Sitting for long periods of time causes stress, and anyone who works sitting down all day can testify to this. Sitting, whether in an office or a vehicle, will eventually cause tightness in the neck, back, and leg muscles. Regular massage helps to prevent or alleviate this symptom of stress.

People who walk all day in their jobs or exercise constantly in a particular way often feel tight and stiff, too. Lifting and pulling can also create a pattern of injury. Whatever the motion, if it is repeated often enough without proper care to form, it may cause muscle damage in the form of spasm or restriction of motion. Changing how we execute a task coupled with exercise and massage helps to prevent further injury and repair old problems.

Think about the stiff neck and shoulders that many folks complain of, or the painful lower back and hips that prevent participation in many events. These are generally attributed to repetitive motion. Every action we take eventually becomes repetitive, simply by the act of living and aging. Often massage can alleviate these painful symptoms.

Recovery from Injury

Once someone has sustained an injury, massage is often helpful during the recovery period and beyond. Areas that have required stitches, upon healing, benefit from massage to assist in preventing scar tissue and releasing adhesions. An adhesion is fibrous tissue that results from an inflammatory process that starts during the healing of separated tissue, as in surgery or an injury. Adhesions can limit muscle movement. Massage stimulates the system allowing the blood to flow effectively to all areas of the body, especially areas of injury. This nourishment helps the healing process, promoting skin and muscle health. The muscles become firmer and the skin becomes more supple with the application of massage. Just think, as you massage your family and friends you are helping them to operate at their best.

When Massage Is Not Called For

Massage is appropriate most of the time; however, there are conditions for which it is not beneficial and is actually contraindicated. Some of these deal with symptoms of disease or particular physical defects, such as abnormal body temperature, inflammation, or vein abnormalities, whereas others deal with certain conditions of the skin. Some are specific disorders while others are more general, yet equally as important.

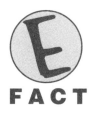

FACT

"Contraindicated" means "inadvisable." For some conditions, massage may be contraindicated entirely, while for others, only certain types of movements or strokes are not recommended. Contraindications in massage protect the giver as well as the receiver.

Abnormal Body Temperature and Inflammation

If someone feels too hot or complains of being feverish, massage is not recommended. A fever is the body's way of fighting off attacks to the immune system. Generally high temperature is a sign to let the body heal itself, without help from you at that moment. Another reason for feeling heat might be inflammation in a particular area. You may be massaging your friend and find an area of the body that is noticeably hotter than anywhere else. Do not work on the hot spot because heat indicates an abnormality. Often such an area will have swelling and sometimes even discoloration. Advise your friend to see a medical practitioner. There are times when you will actually see an open infection that is pus-filled or discolored. Pus is another way the body fights infection by localizing the infection to that area only. Massage could push the infection into the bloodstream, causing a more severe illness, so do not work on the person at all. This infection needs medical attention.

Vein Abnormalities

There are a few conditions affecting the veins for which massage is clearly contraindicated. Varicose veins are the most obvious of these conditions.

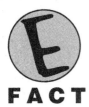

FACT

Varicose veins are caused by the breakdown of the valves that allow blood to pass through the veins in one direction toward the heart. The valves act like inward-opening doors, allowing blood to pass in only one direction, and keeping it from flowing backward. When valve action is faulty, blood flows back through the door, causing a bulge in the vein.

Varicose veins are usually bluish in color, greater than normal in size, and generally bulge out of the lower legs. Sometimes these protruding veins may be painful even without being touched. Varicose veins can be caused by prolonged periods of sitting or standing, when the valves may receive undue stress. Pregnancy and obesity may cause this vein condition as well. Varicose veins may also be inherited. Varicosities can be found anywhere in the legs and should not be touched.

Phlebitis is an inflammation of a vein that can be painful and is generally accompanied by swelling. Often phlebitis can evolve into thrombophlebitis, where a blood clot has formed along the wall of the vein. Massage is clearly contraindicated if this condition exists.

Broken blood vessels should not be massaged, but you can gently massage the area around the vessels.

Skin Conditions

Many skin conditions are not affected by massage. Your concern is with conditions that can be spread over the body of the receiver or to you. The rule of thumb is if the skin is broken, cut, bleeding, or has a rash, do not massage. If the receiver has acne, boils, burns, blisters, eczema, or psoriasis, do not work on the affected area. You may massage other parts of the body but not the affected areas.

Areas affected by sunburn are not to be massaged, either, nor should any parts of the body that have sustained insect stings or bites. If there is contact dermatitis or exposure to poison ivy, oak, or sumac do not massage the body at this time, because this will spread the infection not only on the receiver but to you as well.

Other Conditions

Some disorders require a doctor's go-ahead before you can massage. Folks on any long-term medication or medication for high blood pressure, asthma, nervous disorders, or cancer should check with their medical practitioners before beginning a course of massage. All of these conditions respond well to massage, but a doctor's go-ahead is essential. Once medical consent is given, massage works to support whatever conventional treatment has been arranged.

People with low blood pressure may feel light-headed after a massage; so take care to allow someone with this issue to relax a bit longer on the table, and give a little extra assistance when the person gets up. Heart patients do well with massage once their doctor gives the okay. Although these conditions and disorders do not completely rule out massage, great care must be exercised. If massage is allowed it must be performed gently, and the length of the massage should be reduced. When in doubt do not massage.

Tools Used in Massage

There are a variety of ways to perform a massage. What you need is relatively simple: a flat surface, a private area, and most important, your hands. You can be as fancy or as simple as you wish. Once you have prepared yourself, and know the limitations of your massage partner, you are ready for the next step.

Your Hands

Your hands are your most valuable tools. To start, make sure your nails are cut short and straight across. Always check the length of your nails before beginning a massage. Use a good nail-cleansing brush to keep the nails free of debris.

Always make sure to cleanse your hands carefully with a good soap before you massage. Dr. Bronner's peppermint or lavender liquid soaps are both antibacterial and antifungal. However, any soap will do; use what feels comfortable for your hands and your budget. Start with hot water and soap both hands and forearms well. Rinse first with warm water, and then with cool water to close the pores. Wipe your hands dry with paper towels and dispose of the towels.

Check your hands carefully for any open cuts. Be sure to look at the cuticles as well as the fingertips, and check over your forearms also. Do not work on anyone if you have open, uncovered wounds on your hands or arms. Keep a supply of bandages to cover all tiny cuts, and if you have any open, oozing sores, cuts, or skin disorders, do not work on anyone until these have healed. Keep your hands moisturized, which will leave hands smooth and less likely to chafe or crack. If you are not sure your hands should perform massage, wait until you feel all areas in question have cleared up. However, if you feel strongly that you would like to massage a friend or family member you can always use rubber gloves. Keep a box handy if such an occasion should arise.

A Flat Surface

The floor is one of the flattest surfaces you can find; you just need plenty of cushion to create a firm base. Padding can be a thick piece of foam, or a couple of waffle-type foam mattress pads, or a cotton padded mat, like a futon, or anything that is soft yet pliable. You can use a pile of fleece blankets to form a comfortable cushion, or you can put foam mattress pads in a duvet, roll it up, and take it anywhere. Have massage, will travel!

Working on the floor gives you plenty of room to move around, and gives the receiver the freedom to stretch out. Place pillows under the receiver's knees when working on the front of the body and under the receiver's ankles when working on the back. Make a face rest from rolled towels to hold the receiver's face off the floor and support his or her neck while you are working on the back.

While the floor is a great place to work, some of you may feel stress on your back or your knees as you work. Try kneeling on a pillow to cushion your knees and also give a bit of support to your back. If you find massaging on the floor is not for you, there are other options.

Massage Table

Next to your hands, a massage table is the most important tool you will use if you plan to do a lot of massaging. Working at a table can be much more comfortable than kneeling on the floor over your receiver. Tables can be portable or stationary, homemade or store bought, but any table you decide on should have these features: It should be long enough to accommodate a tall person, wide enough for the receiver's arms to rest easily on the table, and strong enough to support the massage receiver's weight as well as part of your weight as you lean in when working. And make sure the table does not wobble!

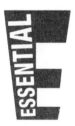

Your massage table should be a comfortable height. To test this, place your hand flat on the top and keep your arm straight. Stand tall with both feet flat on the floor and relax your shoulder. If your hand rests easily, this is a good table for you.

Padding is important too; any table you use should have a good amount of thick, supportive padding to cushion the body. Several layers are best, because this will prevent the receiver from feeling the table and will provide a greater level of support. The idea is to allow the recipient to feel cushioned and supported at the same time.

For home use, a stationary table makes sense, or a table you can easily fold and put away. A good inexpensive choice is to use a sturdy, folding banquet table, if you happen to have one. You can either put down a few layers of foam or fold some blankets to cover the table as the cushion. Foam egg-crate mattress covers work well, as do multilayers of fleece or some other soft blanket.

You can find tables in outlet stores as well as in catalogs, massage magazines, and of course the Internet. It is easy to find a portable table, one that is strong, cushioned, and inexpensive. The beauty of owning a real massage table is the ability to use massage accessories easily.

Accessories for Your Table

A face cradle helps to keep the receiver's head and neck straight when lying facedown, while providing a space for the person to breathe. The face rest is made of foam and is fitted on a circular frame, which is attached to the end of the table. Some face cradles are adjustable, allowing even greater access to the neck. The cradle provides cushion to the face and support for the neck, and adds more length to the table.

Arm supports can either add width or provide a shelf for folks to rest their arms. Side extensions attach to the sides of the table, giving more space for arms to rest slightly away from the body. An arm platform attaches either to the face rest or to the end of the table. This shelf provides a comfortable place for people to rest their arms when they are lying facedown.

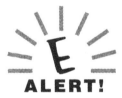

ALERT!

When lying facedown, arms that hang off the table may "fall asleep." You know, that pins and needles feeling! This means the nerve and blood supply is compromised. Whenever you are working on someone in this position make sure the person's arms are resting at his or her sides or supported on a shelf.

If you have made your own table there are ways to provide these features by improvising. Create your own face cradle. Either roll bath towels and curve them in a circle, or buy extra-thick foam and fashion a face rest, covering it with washable fabric that you can remove. Whatever you make, leave room for the face to rest comfortably while letting the neck remain straight. You can create an arm shelf by placing a chair under each side of the table and stacking pillows to the level of the arms. Make certain that the pillows are high enough to rest the arms without stress on the shoulder joints. Experiment with both of these options; try them out to see how they feel.

Massage Chair

Massage can also work if you use a chair. The receiver can sit on a chair, facing the back, resting the arms and head on the back of the chair. The receiver might even sit on a stool, with his or her head and arms resting on a table. The arms are folded with the head resting on the arms; usually a pillow is placed under the arms for support and cushion. You can easily work on the back and neck as well as the arms in this fashion.

A massage chair is a fancier option. It is simple to use and very portable. It is like a mini-table, with a chest support, a headrest, and an armrest. Working with a chair gives you access only to the back, neck, and arms, but fortunately these are often the areas folks like to have you work on. You can perform a massage anywhere with this type of setup. Generally chair massage is given while the receiver is fully clothed so you could even massage your friends at work.

Bolsters for Support

Pillows, wedges, and circular bolsters are all supportive cushions that you will want to acquire. These will provide welcome support whether the receiver is lying facedown or on his or her back. Neck cushions come in a variety of shapes, or you can make your own using rolled towels. Simply roll a thick bath towel into a tight cylinder, and slip it under the back of the neck. This will provide support and cushion while allowing the person's head to rest comfortably on the table.

A pillow placed under the knees helps to take pressure off the back when the person is lying face up. Facedown, a pillow under the ankles will provide support and relieve the back. A wedge-shaped pillow is a versatile tool to place in the narrow edge under the knees, or under the ankles. A wedge can be slipped under the back as well.

Clean Linens

Acquire a good supply of cotton sheets that you use only for massage. Flannel sheets provide extra warmth and feel comforting in the cool months. White sheets are the easiest to keep in good condition because they can be bleached many times without appearing stained or discolored. Twin-size sheets are the perfect size. Be sure to cover all your pillows with clean pillowcases each time you give a massage. These should be cotton, too.

Bath sheet towels make great covers if they are large and soft. These provide effective coverage and can be used to drape around the receiver getting on and off the table. Towels usually can withstand being washed in bleach, too.

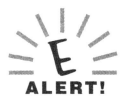

ALERT!

All sheets, towels, and pillowcases must be changed with each receiver. Never use the same linens! Wash everything in detergent and bleach and dry in a hot dryer. Wash massage linens separately; do not mix with your personal laundry.

Use lightweight yet warm blankets to provide extra warmth and cover. Fleece is an ideal weight for the cool months: easy to clean, very warm, yet not too heavy. A light cotton blanket or spread will work in the hotter months if extra cover is needed. All fabrics should be washable.

Soothing Music

Massage music is everywhere. Any store that sells music will have a variety of relaxation recordings. Look for music that is instrumental, featuring soft healing sounds. Music for massage, yoga, meditation, and energy healing provides the soothing rhythm appropriate for bodywork. Some folks prefer total silence, practicing in-the-moment mindfulness while they receive the massage. Always check to see what your recipient likes.

Gentle Lights

Natural light provides the best atmosphere for massage. If the room you work in has plenty of natural light take advantage of it. Use curtains or blinds that allow the light to filter in while still providing privacy. But not all rooms where you massage will have the advantage of natural lighting. Soft, clear lights work best: either small table lamps or a floor lamp placed away from the work area. Do not use harsh, glaring lamps or overhead lights.

Appropriate Draping

Privacy in massage is extremely important. It is essential that the receiver feels safe and secure. Let the receiver know that you recognize and respect his or her vulnerability, and that you are honored by his or her trust. It is easy to provide a secure cover; a flat twin sheet is very effective, as is a bath sheet or beach towel. Uncover only the part of the body you are working on; all else should be protected by the sheet or towel. Some folks like to keep their arms out—whatever feels comfortable is fine.

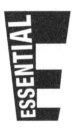

There are different stages of undress, depending upon the level of comfort the receiver feels. Let people know it is up to them whether they wish to be completely naked under the cover, or keep their underwear on or even some of their clothes. The state of undress is a matter the individual should decide.

For some, getting undressed will be done in private. If the receiver is going to disrobe in the same room where you will be giving the massage, leave him or her alone at this time. Give the receiver a towel or robe to put on until you can help him or her onto the table or down on the mat. Often folks will already be under the covers when you return; others may need your help. Of course, if you are working on your spouse or significant partner, different rules apply! And there is always the friend who is a massage veteran, who is usually undressed and on the table before you can even leave the room to wash your hands.

Oils, Creams, or Powders

Using a lubricant allows your hands to glide easily when performing the massage strokes. There are many different types of lubrication, each with a distinct purpose for use in a specific way. Experiment with a variety of products to find what you like best.

Whether you use oil or cream when you massage will depend on what you like as well as what the recipient prefers. Some people like the feel of a heavy cream sinking into their skin while others adore the feeling of warm oil as their skin drinks the healing properties. Some conditions respond better with the use of an essential oil applied in small diluted quantities. Whatever you use, remember, what is important is how good the massage and the products you use feel on the receiver.

Using Oils

Oils provide a smooth, friction-free medium that allows you to massage large areas easily. There are many different types of oils: some are natural vegetable- and plant-based oils; others are essential oils; while others are made from nuts or seeds. Choose oils that nourish the skin, rather than oils that contain alcohol or mineral oil, because these rob the skin of nutrients.

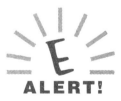

Always check with your receiver to see if she has any known allergy or skin condition. Often folks are aware of what products they can or cannot use. Discuss the contents of the massage medium before applying it. When in doubt use a hypoallergenic product, or ask the recipient to provide the lubricant.

Make sure you are aware of your receiver's tolerance to fragrance and nut-based products. A good basic oil is natural jojoba oil, which can be used alone or with essential oils. It does not spoil and generally does not cause any reactions. Another bonus is that jojoba does not stain the sheets or your clothing.

Using Creams and Lotions

Creams and lotions are thicker than oil, with less gliding ability. Lotion absorbs easily into the skin, whereas cream needs more rubbing before the skin soaks it up. Both of these massage mediums are easy to use and are less greasy than many oils. Cream may be easier for you to use when you want to work deep in the muscle. Cream and lotion are both good to use on the face or any area where oil is not preferred. Cream also works well on regions that are hairy, like calves and backs, because the hands are able to glide easily and the cream keeps the areas moist.

Using Powder

Powder reduces the friction when massaging, but it is not as good as cream, lotion, or oil. Powder is good to use on oily skin or when the recipient does not want any oil or cream on his or her body. A receiver with excessive body hair or an eruptive skin condition, like acne, is better served with the use of powder. The best powder to use is a cornstarch- or other natural-base powder made from plants or grains, because these are less likely to clog the pores.

Whatever you use to provide lubrication, always apply the medium to your hands first and then to the body. Do not put the oil, lotion, cream, or powder directly on the body because the cool sensation will be jarring to the recipient. Pour, shake, or scoop the lubricant into your hands, gently warming it first, and then apply it. You can have fun trying the different massage media, experimenting with everything, deciding what you like best, and practicing on yourself and others. Ⓔ

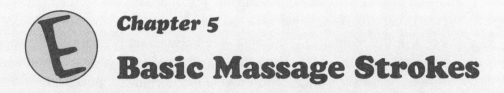

Chapter 5

Basic Massage Strokes

To begin any massage, first consider the quality of your touch. You have prepared your space and yourself; now it is time to practice sensitive contact and learn how to enter into another's sphere with confidence and compassion. You will learn to create an atmosphere of comfort and trust, conveying your sense of integrity and caring to the receiver. Your hands will become involved in healing as you practice and then perform different massage strokes on others and yourself.

First Touch

The initial touch in massage sets the tone for continued relaxation. As with any touch therapy, it is essential to create an atmosphere of harmony that allows for total flow and release. First, give the person receiving the massage a moment to relax as you become aware of the rhythm of his or her breath. Watch for steady, relaxed breathing as you approach the recipient.

Be sure the receiver is arranged comfortably on the table. Certain areas of the recipient's body may need added support, including knees, ankles, head, and neck. Remember, you can use a variety of pillows, towels, wedges, or bolsters to provide comfort and support during the session. Place these props under the knees or the head and neck if the person is lying face up; if the recipient is lying facedown, place a bolster under the ankles.

Draping with sheets or towels is important for warmth and security, whether your receiver prefers to be clothed or not. Some recipients prefer to receive massage wearing underwear or athletic shorts and tops. Whatever a person feels comfortable with is correct for that person. You can use cotton or fleece blankets for additional warmth if needed.

Where to Start

There is no right place to begin a massage. Where to start on the body will become your choice as you grow into the art of applying massage. Some people like to begin on the back because it provides a large surface for the beginning strokes. Others prefer to start with a face or foot massage. Wherever you begin is the best starting point for you.

The following examples deal initially with the back. The back is always a safe area to begin because it is a nonthreatening zone with ample room to apply a variety of strokes, and it provides a broad canvas to create your masterpiece. The following discussion explains how to use the back as your starting point.

Establish a Connection

With your partner lying facedown, stand to the side, letting your body become comfortable with your position. Place both hands gently on the covered body, letting your still, quiet touch flow into the receiver. Let your hands rest in this peaceful position, encouraging deeper relaxation. This announcement of safe touch informs the recipient of the giver's intent. So begins your journey with informed touch.

As your hands gently rest on the recipient, breathe slowly and evenly, silently influencing the breathing of the receiver. Move one hand to the nape of the neck and the other to the small of the back, drawing an invisible energy line. Perhaps you are guided to let both hands rest gently on the upper back, creating an energy connection there. The idea here is to allow yourself to become aware of your intuitive sense. Your hands are the tools that will guide you through this process, signaling areas of stress and discomfort.

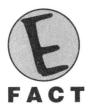

FACT

Intuition is defined as the act of knowing without rational thought. Our sense of intuition allows us to instinctively know or feel something without thinking, and is an aspect of our senses that we use every day.

The first touch opens the pathway of communication between the body you are working on and your hands. See if you feel tension in the body under your hands. Is the back tight? How does the neck feel? Let the eyes within your hands reveal what the skin is relaying. Once you feel comfortable with your assessment, you are ready to begin.

Stroking Touch (Effleurage)

Stroking is the first general movement in massage. Stroking is just what it seems—long, defined moves that glide along the skin's surface. The technical name for this movement is effleurage (pronounced ef-flu-rahj). Effleurage is a smooth, gliding stroke that is employed in a variety of techniques.

Effleurage touch should be a light, soft movement as you begin to apply oil and soften the muscles. Your initial smooth gliding strokes allow you to cover a large area, introducing touch in a soft, acceptable style.

Effleurage is applied using your hands, fingers, and at times your forearm. As you stroke the skin tissue you affect circulation and stimulate the lymphatic system. Once the recipient's muscles are relaxed, your touch should become deep, penetrating work, reaching down into the areas of greatest resistance.

Effleurage strokes should be applied with lighter pressure as you move down the body and deeper pressure as you move up the body, imitating the flow of blood. By using lighter pressure going away from the heart and deeper pressure coming toward the heart you will assist in proper circulation throughout the body. By encouraging circulation you help to clear toxins and supply nourishment to all the organs of the body.

Practicing Gentle Effleurage

Imagine the back as a clean canvas waiting for you to paint a picture. Stand behind the receiver's head, so that you are looking down along the recipient's back. Using the oil you and your partner have selected, hold a small amount in your hands, letting the oil receive your body's warmth. Rub your hands together, coating them with oil, and place both hands on the back between the shoulders. Move your hands simultaneously down the back on either side of the spine, spreading the oil.

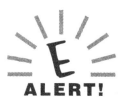
ALERT!

Never press on the spine! If you gently run your fingers down the spine you will feel the bony vertebrae that protect the spinal cord. You should also feel the muscles that attach to and support the spine. To avoid injury of this sensitive area, always work the area next to the spine, not on top of it.

Keeping your hands on the back, move down near the waistline; then pull the hands back up toward the shoulders, still gliding. Continue to make long strokes down and long strokes back up, covering the entire back. It will seem as though you are drawing half moons on the back. Let your body move in as you stroke downward and lean back as you pull up. Use a flat, open hand, keeping contact with the skin as much as possible. The strokes should continue to be smooth and gliding, eventually becoming deeper as the muscles begin to relax. Let yourself feel the skin responding to your touch. Each circuit around the back allows deeper penetration. Trust what your hands are telling you about the skin underneath.

Fingers Can Be Used, Too

Some areas of the body are too small to accommodate your entire open hand when applying effleurage. When you massage the face, for example, use just your fingers to bring long, sliding strokes to the skin. The fingers gently glide along the surface of the face, bringing relaxation to a tense jaw or forehead.

The feather stroke is another form of effleurage. This involves letting the fingers act like fluttering feathers as you lightly stroke the surface of the body, using just your fingertips or your entire hand. Feathering gently calms the nerve endings, which is a great finishing touch to the part of the body you're working on. Gently feathering the fingers along the back is sometimes used as a transitional move from the back to another part of the body.

The Electromagnetic Field

Another form of effleurage is called aura stroking, which is extremely relaxing to the receiver. Here the hand does not touch the body, but rather it strokes from above. Using both hands placed together with thumbs touching, slowly and smoothly glide your hands just above the back. Standing at the side of the body, begin at the waist and glide your hands up the back, beginning in the center, making sure you are not actually touching the body. Come back to the waist and work up and down one side completely; move to the other side of the body and glide up and down again. Repeat your gliding movements three times each. Pay attention to the feeling in your palms. You may feel heat, or coolness, or a sense of energy rushing through them.

Scientists are still studying the electromagnetic energy field, or aura, found surrounding the body. Working with this subtle body of energy allows us to influence the body, mind, and spirit of the receiver in a profoundly healing capacity.

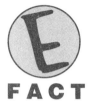

In the late 1900s a Russian scientist, S. D. Kirlian, developed a scientific method of photography, later called Kirlian photography, that documents the electromagnetic field around living beings. Today known as electrophotography, or Kirlian photography, it allows us to discern the colors in the auric field around the subjects' head, feet, and hands. Use of Kirlian photography as a diagnostic tool is growing.

Kneading Strokes (Petrissage)

Kneading, or petrissage, is an effective technique to use after effleurage. Effleurage has softened the muscles, and now the body is prepared for you to go in deeper. In petrissage, you actually lift the skin and muscle, and apply a wringing, pinching, squeezing, rolling, or pressing movement. Simply put, it is a kneading movement that moves the deeper tissues of the body. This technique works to stretch the muscle, increase blood flow, and break up scar tissue.

FIGURE 5-1

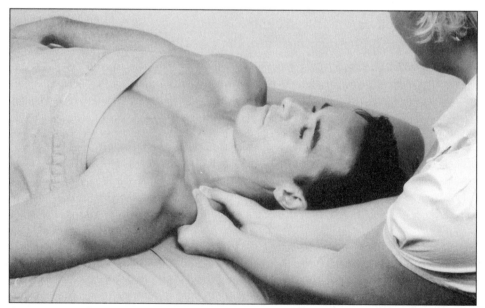

▲ Deep muscle kneading.

Petrissage can be used over large areas of the body as well as on small sections. Use both hands on broad surfaces and one hand on smaller regions. At times only the palm or fingers and thumb are used, as illustrated in **FIGURE 5-1**, where the fingers and thumbs alone knead deeply into the back and shoulder muscles. As the grasped or pressed muscle is released, firmly press on the area and move smoothly on to the next area in a circular motion.

Petrissage is an important technique, meaning this is one to practice, practice, and practice. The rhythm of movement is important here. Remember to move not only your hands but your body as well, tailoring the amount of pressure by the rhythm of your motion.

An Exercise in Kneading

Practice the basic movement of kneading on the back of your massage partner. Stand to the right side of the body, and place your hands on the left area of the back. Start with the lower back and grasp a handful of flesh (the skin and the muscle beneath it) in your left hand, lifting and squeezing without pinching. Use your entire hand with your fingers overlapping onto the flesh and your thumb a bit in front. Let your hand move in a circular motion.

Bring your right hand into play now, grasping another handful of flesh and repeating the same movement, holding the skin and muscle while moving the hand in a circular motion. Both hands should move in the same direction, firmly grasping the skin and moving in a slight circular motion. Move your body side to side as you perform this movement. Slide the flesh from your right hand toward your left and move your right hand up a bit along the back. The left hand grasps the flesh released by the right, and the right hand picks up a new section.

Continue to roll, grasp, and pinch the flesh as you work up to the shoulder. Switch sides and work up the back again, using the same technique.

Remember to move your body in time with the motion of your hands. If your hands become tired, you are not using your *body* to apply the pressure, which is where the effort should come from. Also, check to see how your hands are positioned on the recipient's body—if your wrists are bent, unbend them. If you tend to reach too far across the body, move your position so you are not off balance.

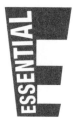

A good way to practice the kneading technique on your own is to knead some dough, either bread dough or play dough. Pay attention to how you must move your body in order to really see the dough change shape and texture. Practice all the different techniques of kneading while you work the dough.

Rolling Technique

Rolling is kneading only the top layers of tissue with the thumb and fingers. Stay on the left side of the body, with your hands resting on the same side of the back. Your right hand is closest to the waist and your left hand next to it. Using your fingers and thumbs, grasp a small amount of skin and gently roll it back and forth. Your fingers push the skin toward your thumbs, and your thumbs roll the skin back to your fingers. Continue this back-and-forth movement as you move up along the left side of the spine to the shoulders. Return to the waist on this same side and roll up again. Repeat as many times as needed to cover this side of the back. Move over to the right side and practice rolling there.

Wringing Technique

Wringing is a form of petrissage best used on the arms and legs. Imagine wringing out your favorite shirt: One hand twists one way and the other hand twists in the opposite direction. This alternate back-and-forth movement is gentle, yet deep. Use just enough oil to allow an easy, sliding motion as you wring up and down.

Let's practice on the arms. It is easiest to apply this technique with the receiver lying face up. Help your partner turn over by holding the drape up and slightly away, letting him or her turn freely. Tuck the drape back in, leaving one arm uncovered. Standing to the side of the body, grasp the uncovered arm and firmly wring back and forth, moving up the arm from the elbow to the shoulder.

Bend the arm at the elbow, grasp under the wrist with both hands, and wring up and down the forearm. Use firm steady pressure as you move toward the elbow, and a lighter touch as you move back toward the wrist. Finish at the elbow, wringing two or three more times. Rest the receiver's forearm on the table and cover this arm. Move to the other side and repeat.

Friction Strokes

Friction is a form of massage that moves the top layers of tissue over the deeper layers, causing the deeper muscle to be stimulated. Applied after effleurage and petrissage, this massage stroke allows the muscles to generate heat as they are rubbed together. Friction is good for releasing tight muscles, loosening scar tissue, as well as increasing circulation. Friction around joint areas reaches the underlying tissue effectively and may soothe aching joints. Use your fingers, the heels of your palms, and occasionally just your thumbs to apply friction, which can be fast-paced or slow and deep. Generally the brisk style requires more oil, whereas the deeper movement needs very little lubricant.

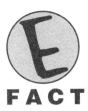

FACT

If the movement is a gliding, sliding type of motion, make sure to use enough oil. Deep-tissue work needs very little oil, because too much may cause slipping from the area. Dry skin may need more oil, and so will elderly skin. Someone with a lot of body hair may need lotion *and* oil. Experiment!

The use of friction strokes in massage illustrates the body's ability to heal itself. The benefits of applying friction techniques are numerous. For example, friction techniques can . . .

- Stretch and soften tissue.
- Break up scar tissue.
- Increase heat in the body.
- Increase the metabolic rate.

- Promote exchange of interstitial fluid (fluid between the cells and blood vessels).
- Increase circulation to skin.
- Increase circulation to joints.

Practicing Basic Friction Strokes

Ask your massage partner to return to the facedown position, and tuck the drape in at the waist as you prepare again to work on the back. Stand at the head of the table looking down on the receiver's back. Taking a little bit of oil in your hands, rub your palms together and feel the heat from this small bit of friction. Place your hands on the shoulders, palms flat on the body, fingers close together. Lean in a bit and push your right hand down the back along the right edge of the spine. When this hand reaches the waist, push your left hand down along the left edge. At the same time, bring your right hand back up to the shoulder.

Continue to work in this fashion, pressing one hand down as the other pulls back. Feel the heat under your hands as the friction begins to heat up the muscles. Use your body to apply the pressure, creating a back-and-forth rhythm. This form of friction massage on the back is moving in the direction of the muscle fibers.

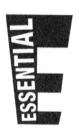

The movement of your body is essential to the success of your strokes. Remember to always move your body as you work with massage. Do not be afraid to move! Move back and forth or side to side depending upon the area you are working on as well as the technique you are employing.

Circular Friction

Circular friction is exactly what it sounds like—friction applied in a circular fashion. To practice this technique, position yourself at the head of the table. Let your hands rest palm down at the shoulders, fingers together pointing down toward the waist. Lift the palms of your hands up so your fingers are facing down with the pads resting on the back. Then move your body forward and press in with your fingers.

Feel the muscles underneath as they give in to the pressure. Let your fingers rest in the small groove or indentation you have created. Slowly begin to make small circles, moving the flesh, not the fingers, and feel the tissues under the skin move. Bring your fingers up a bit onto the surface of the skin and make circles again, with no pressure. Press in and cause friction. Feel the difference? When you apply pressure you are working the muscle under the surface of the skin. When you let up on the pressure you are working only the top layer of the skin.

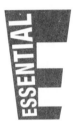

To help you understand the feeling of friction, first work on a clothed body. With your hands on the receiver's back, apply a little pressure and circle on one spot with your fingertips. The shirt doesn't move, but the skin underneath does. This will simulate the feeling of one layer of skin moving beneath the other.

Cross Friction

Muscle fibers are formed in bundles of fibers that all run in the same direction. Cross-fiber strokes work across the muscle tissue rather than in the direction of the muscle fiber. This is a deeper movement for which you can use your fingers, thumbs, and sometimes the heels of your palm. Place your fingers on the area of stress, and move them in a walking manner across the area and back again. The pressure from your fingers causes the top layer of skin to move the under layer, without gliding, just as in the circular technique. Of course, most of the pressure comes from the movement of your body, as you move back and forth or side to side.

For deeper access, place one hand on top of the other. While the bottom hand performs the crossing stroke, the palm is moving across the skin with friction as the top hand applies more pressure. This technique allows for deep penetration to a painful area.

Tapping Strokes (Tapotement)

Tapotement, or tapping, is a percussive technique used to produce stimulation, treating the body as though it is a drum. The movement is a steady, even beat that produces a flush to the skin, a feeling of well-being, and a sensation of renewed energy. There are many different forms of tapping that are created by different positions of the hands and fingers. Some of the most popular forms are hacking, cupping, slapping, tapping, and chopping. Always keep your hands loose from the wrist, including the fingers and thumbs, as shown in the example of chopping in **FIGURE 5-2**.

FIGURE 5-2

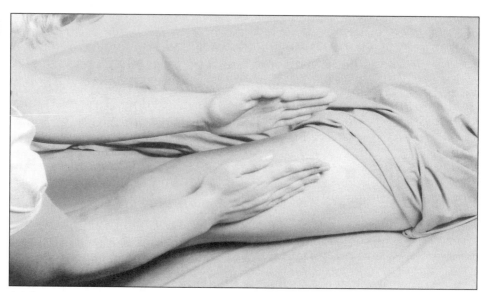

▲ Chopping technique.

Practice for a moment relaxing your hands. Sit or stand and shake out your hands, letting them become loose. Your hands and wrists will flap back and forth, your fingers will hit each other, and your thumbs will do their own thing. Let your arms fall to the side and relax from the shoulders. Allow everything to become loose and free.

Next, practice drumming. Place your fingers on a hard surface, like a table, and start out slowly. Tap the table one finger at a time in progression, creating a smooth pattern. Let your fingers be easy and gentle as you move into a steady beat. You can use your thumbs to brace your hands as your fingers do the tapping. Pick up the pace; see how the table begins to talk back to you? When your fingers feel a slight pain, ease up the pressure but continue the beat.

Continue to experiment with tapping, making your own composition. The idea is to provide an even, comfortable experience that will stimulate while adding to the overall feeling of renewal. Tapping should not be so hard that it hurts! Rather than tapping harder, let the fingers all tap together; this will feel more intense.

Still on the hard surface, let your hands form the chopping position in **FIGURE 5-2**, but this time let your fingers remain loose. Chop your hands slowly on the table (not too hard or it will be painful) and pick up the pace as you become confident with this move.

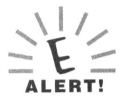
ALERT!

Massage therapists must be ever conscious of their bodies. Proper positioning is crucial to your ability to work, as well as to the overall health of your joints, connective tissues, and the muscles in your hands. Practice keeping your arms and hands relaxed but not overly extended or flexed.

Practice drumming and chopping on your legs so you become comfortable with the feel. Use an open palm with your fingers slightly cupped and gently slap on your legs. Feel the slight vacuum caused by the curved palm. Now flatten your palm, straighten your fingers, and slap your legs. This feels different because the fingers do more of the slapping. Practice these two moves on your legs and find out what feels good and what is too much.

Lastly, close your hands into very loose fists and pound lightly on your legs. This pounding or hacking is good for very large muscles such as those on the thighs or the back (but not near the waistline). Try this on yourself: Using your loosely closed fist, pound on your thighs with the sides of your hands; then turn your fists and rapidly beat a staccato rhythm on your thighs. Feel how the different ways of pounding stimulate your leg muscles? In massage, we call this hacking. It also works well on hamstring muscles, found on the back of the thighs, as demonstrated in **FIGURE 5-3**.

FIGURE 5-3

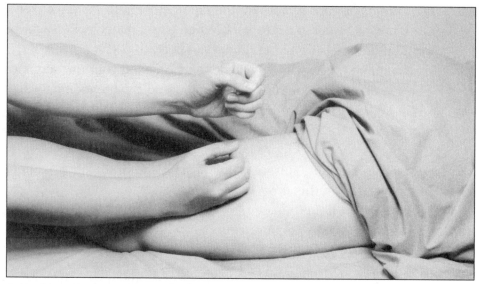

▲ Hacking the hamstring muscles.

Become aware of the different feelings these tapping techniques deliver. After trying them all out on yourself, practice on your massage partner. Ask for feedback, continuously checking the comfort level of your receiver.

Other Basic Strokes

Vibrating, shaking, and rocking are massage techniques that produce relaxation or stimulation depending upon the delivery. These movements can produce a soothing effect to the nerve endings of the skin. Of the three, vibration is perhaps the most difficult to learn.

Massage with Vibration

When using a vibration stroke properly, your body will actually tremble. To get started, place your hand on your receiver's back. Bring your hand up so that only the fingers, mostly the fingertips, have contact on the skin. Let your entire arm shake from the fingers to the shoulder. Stiffen your muscles so that this shivering, trembling motion flows down into your fingertips. This is hard to do, so be patient. Once you have the trembling, shaking, shivering, vibrating movement under control, sustain the vibrations as you drag your fingertips, feeling the muscles underneath begin to loosen. The object of vibration is to free the muscles as you continue to move along the surface.

Shaking the Muscles

Shaking helps to loosen tight muscles. You can place your hand flat on a large muscle and gently shake the area. Or you can literally pick up an arm or leg and very gently shake it to free up tension. Lift the arm of your receiver straight out from the table and gently shake it, taking care not to pull or twist the arm. The muscles will loosen from the shoulder down to the fingertips. Another way to shake out an arm is to gently glide your fingers between your receiver's fingers, using your other hand to help you secure your fingers, as shown in **FIGURE 5-4**. Once the hand is securely held, you may stretch the arm up and out without any help from the receiver and shake it while your fingers are interlocked.

FIGURE 5-4

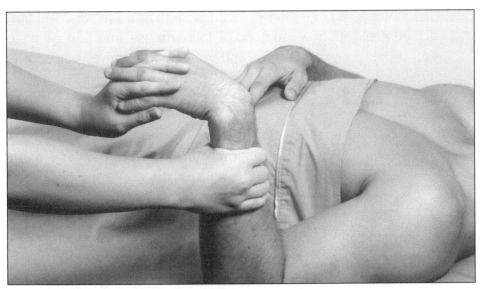

▲ Interlock fingers to stretch the arm.

Another form of shaking is applied directly to the muscle. Place your hands on the receiver's back, using one hand to hold the back in place while the other does the work. With the working hand shake the muscle underneath. This is a very subtle move, and you will need to pay attention.

Rocking the Body

Rocking is a fun technique that brings comfort to you and to the recipient. With the recipient lying on the table facedown, place one hand on the recipient's shoulder and the other on the waist. Gently begin to rock your body back and forth. As you do, your receiver will begin to rock also. Pull and push back and forth to establish your rhythm. Once you have a good rock going the body will almost rock itself.

Experiment with rocking. As you rock the body, start to pick up a bit of speed. Once the body is rocking well, push but do not pull back, and let the body rock back on its own. An uptight body will resist rocking whereas a relaxed body will flow. Your goal is to create the natural ebb and flow from the rhythm of the receiver. Work with this for a while; try different speeds and different positions.

All of the strokes and techniques discussed in this chapter are the basic ones used in massage. Practice them and see what you like best. Experiment with how much oil or lotion to use, and find out which works best for you. Have fun and remember to move your body and exercise your hands!

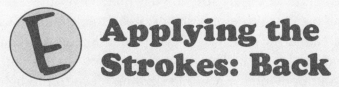 Applying the Strokes: Back

It is exciting to learn massage! The specific strokes are applied in a variety of ways to various parts of the body. The following chapters will take you through a basic full-body massage. You will follow a simple pattern that allows you to massage the entire body or parts of the body. The best part of being able to actually perform massage will be your own improvising. Once you have mastered the strokes and the easy pattern, the fun of adding and changing begins.

Working the Back

Once you and your receiver have prepared for the massage as explained in Chapter 4, and the receiver is lying comfortably facedown on the massage surface, stand at the side of the table, place your hands on the receiver's covered back, and let your hands rest lightly on its flat broad surface. Gently spread your hands over the back, as though pressing the cover free of wrinkles. Lean into the back using your body to create a rocking type of movement, letting your hands move down and up the back. The movement of your hands and the movement of your body create a subtle rhythm. Move to the head of the table and lean in with your body as your hands travel down the back toward the waist. Move backward a bit with your body, and your hands move back toward the shoulders.

Again at the side of the table, fold back the cover and tuck it in around the receiver's hips. Apply oil to your hands and, with your hands flat, gently stroke down either side of the spine and back up again with long, gliding effleurage strokes. **FIGURE 6-1** shows the proper position for your hands.

FIGURE 6-1

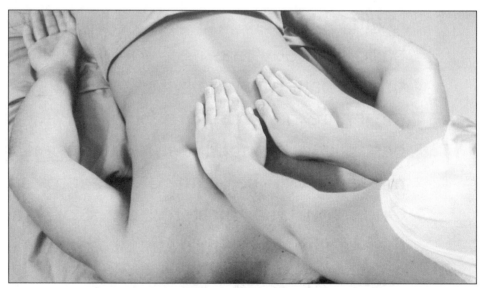

▲ Long gliding stroke on the entire back.

Remain at the receiver's head while you perform these effleurage movements six times. Next, move to the right side of the body and effleurage from the waist up to the shoulders and back down to the waist, applying more oil if needed. Your hands will push up along either side of the spine in strong sweeping strokes, then down along the outer back. Repeat these movements six times.

Now let your hands rest flat on the wings of the shoulder blades, or the scapula. Both hands will be pointing in toward the spine. Move your hands in a circular motion over this area, on either side of the spine. Again use your body as you perform this technique, rocking toward the body and away as you complete the circles. Six circles usually will do.

Repeat this using your fingers, pressing in along the bony landmarks of the shoulder. Here you will make a smaller circular motion, actually resting one hand on top of the other and letting the weight of the resting hand move the tips of your fingers deeper, as you can see in **FIGURE 6-2**.

FIGURE 6-2

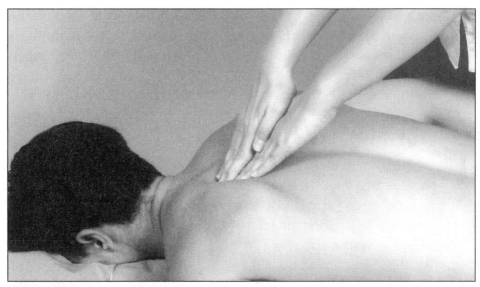

▲ Circular stroke on the shoulder blades.

Deep on the Shoulders

Move your hands up to the shoulders, bringing both hands to the left shoulder first. Using your fingers, stroke along the top edge of the shoulder blade from the spine out to the end of the shoulder. Actually press in with your fingers, and gently pull toward your body off the shoulder. Stretch the skin in the same manner on the right side. Next, lay your hands to one side of the spine, pressing your fingers in as you pull down along the edge of the shoulder to the top of the arm. Repeat at least three times.

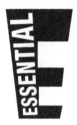

Always make sure you have enough oil to move easily along the skin. The amount of oil you use should allow smooth, steady strokes on every part of the body. If you use too much oil you will slip and slide; too little and you will limit your movement. Remember to spread the oil with gliding effleurage strokes.

Deep effleurage in this manner along the entire top of the back, tracing the shoulder from the spine to the arm, pressing in with your palm and stretching. Continue to move down along the side of the spine, pressing in and stretching out every stroke to the edge of the body. Cover the entire back in this fashion, working on both sides of the spine. Stand on either the right or the left, depending upon which side is comfortable for you.

From the Side

Stand on either side of the body, letting your arms reach across the back, resting your hands along the side of the back. This area is known as the oblique muscles. Using the kneading petrissage stroke, lift, roll, and gently squeeze along the entire side from the hip up to the underarm as shown in **FIGURE 6-3**.

Be sure to assess the amount of pressure you are using as you lift and hold the skin. Repeat this movement back and forth along the side, eventually moving onto the back's surface. Continue to make imaginary lines from the hip up to the shoulder, steadily rolling and squeezing the skin until you reach the line of the spine. Switch sides and repeat. Both hands alternate lifting and kneading back and forth, following the pattern you have already established.

FIGURE 6-3

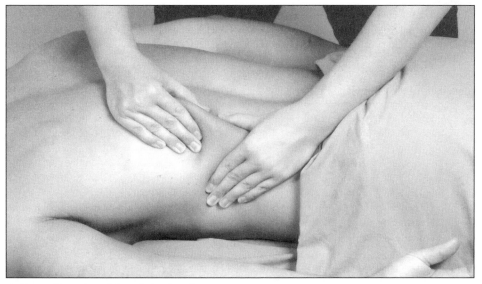

▲ Kneading the side of the back.

Pressing the Upper Shoulders

Move back to the head of the table and place both your palms in the nook of the receiver's shoulder just where it touches the neck. Press in with both palms, pushing and stretching along the top of the shoulder, the trapezius muscle, to the top of the arm, the deltoid muscle. Repeat this three to six times, pressing in firmly as you push down and stretch to the side. Check with the receiver to make sure the pressure is appropriate.

Using the Forearm

While still at the head of the table, move toward the receiver's right shoulder, and place your bent forearm on the receiver's back. Your elbow should rest alongside the spine as shown in **FIGURE 6-4**.

Gently move the forearm down the right side of the back in a long sweeping motion. Using the forearm allows a deeper, longer stroke, covering a broader area. Move your body in as you glide along. When you reach just above the buttocks, known as the gluteal muscles, glide back up again. Continue for three or four times before moving to the left side, and repeat.

Do not use your elbow to press in, because this can cause damage to the underlying muscles. Also, you do not need to press hard; the motion of your arm and the movement of your body allow deep penetration without a lot of effort. Remember to check the receiver's comfort level.

FIGURE 6-4

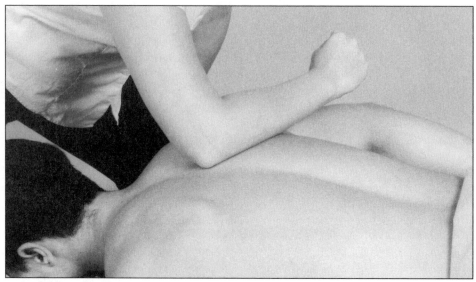

▲ Forearm sweeping down the back.

Easy Stroking

Place your hands flat on the left side of the spine near the base and gently stroke up to the shoulder and back down to the tops of the buttocks. Use long sweeping strokes as you lean into the body. You are smoothing out the back muscles, so you want to use gentle, firm touch to encourage the muscles to relax. Move to the right side of the body and again effleurage down along the spine and up again. Remember, these are smooth, rhythmic strokes applied with the flat of your hand as you glide along the back. Glide your hands down and back in a half-horseshoe type of movement on each side of the back.

The Neck and Back of the Arms

Where you finish on the back suggests the transition you will make to either the neck or the back of the arms. If you are standing in front of the head the logical movement is to the neck, whereas if you end standing at the side of the body you will probably begin with the arms. This time you ended by the head, so you will continue on with the neck.

Using your finger pads, start at the base of the neck, making tiny circles up into the base of the skull. You do not work on the bony spine region of course. Small squiggly movements can be made up and down the neck using very light pressure. Circle the entire back of the neck and then move up into the space on either side of the skull base. This is known as the occipital area, and is covered by a group of muscles. Hold your fingers in at the notches just under the base of the skull right below the ears (to the right and left of the spinal cord), pull in slightly, and you will feel the muscles relax with the easy stretch you are applying. This area holds a great amount of tension so do not be afraid to press and hold gently to the count of five. Lastly, bring your fingers to the side of the neck and, using a slight pinch-and-roll motion, move up the side of the neck back into the occipitals. Press down and away along the ridge of the neck to the shoulders in transition to massaging the arms.

FIGURE 6-5

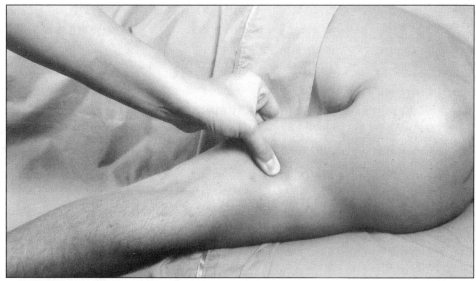

▲ Kneading stroke on the back of the upper arm.

To begin massaging the arms, stand on the right side of the body with both hands resting near the top of the arm. Rest your left hand on the receiver's shoulder blade and your right hand on the deltoid area. Keep your left hand resting slightly while your right hand holds the arm and glides down in a smooth holding motion. Repeat this three times from the shoulder to the fingertips.

Using both hands now wring along the entire arm from the shoulder to the wrist; repeat this three times, down the arm and up again. Now using your right hand, lift the muscles of the upper arm and knead with a lift-pinch-roll movement starting at the shoulder and moving to the wrist. At the elbow carefully and gently let your thumb and index finger make gentle circles around the bone, passing on to the forearm. Continue to knead with the lift-pinch-and-roll motion, using your thumb and index finger as shown in **FIGURE 6-5**.

Gently pass your hand along the entire arm three times from shoulder to wrist and repeat these moves on the left side, using the left hand predominantly.

The Lower Body

With your receiver still lying facedown, tuck the cover around his or her shoulders to keep the upper body warm. Lift the cover from the left leg and tuck the cover between the legs with the loose end over the opposite thigh, as you can see in **FIGURE 6-6**.

Apply oil to your hands, and starting at the buttock use both hands to make smooth gliding strokes down the leg, making sure the leg has enough oil. Move back and forth three or four times. With both hands, wring all along the leg from just below the buttock to the ankle and back up again, three or four times. Now, starting from the top of the thigh, with two hands lift and squeeze the skin down the leg and back, twice. You can see how to hold your hands in **FIGURE 6-7**.

Come up to the hip and, using the pads of your fingers, circle over the entire buttock on this side, firmly. Your fingers are looking for sore areas, which the receiver may have already indicated; if not you will find them. Sore areas generally show resistance with tight muscles, which respond well to massage.

FIGURE 6-6

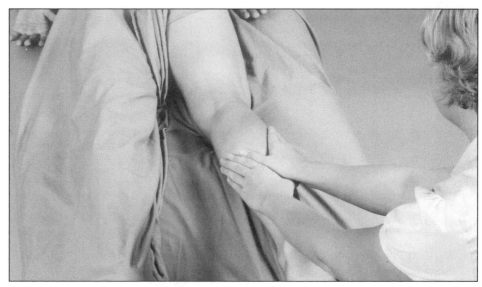

▲ Tuck the cover over the other leg.

FIGURE 6-7

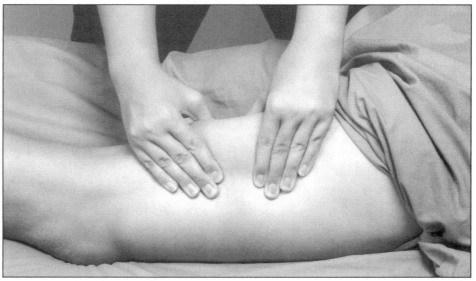

▲ Kneading stroke down the back of the leg.

Don't forget the side of the hip. With your left hand at the side of the hip, alternate between palm and fingers in a deep circular movement. Work around the entire hip area up onto the back of the buttock as well.

Circle and knead where possible; this will release a great deal of muscle tension.

Now stand by the receiver's feet and lift the left foot with both your hands. Keeping the knee bent, cup the underside of the foot with your palms while your thumbs make circular motions on the sole. Slowly lower the foot, gliding your hands to the back of the calf. Use all your fingers to circle up to the knee. Gently circle around the back of the knee, but do not apply pressure.

Bring your hands back to the ankle, and very lightly circle around the ankle area; this is a sensitive spot that does not need a great amount of pressure. Using all your fingers press in across the entire calf area horizontally. Slowly walk and press your fingers across the entire calf using a kneading motion, and work your way up to the knee. After you have worked the calf area sideways, begin again at the ankle region and walk and press up the calf to the back of the knee using vertical lines.

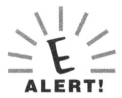

ALERT!

The depression at the ankle is a tender area, and so is the entire area behind the knee. Both of these areas must be worked with a light touch. If the receiver has varicose veins do not work directly on the veins; rather, massage carefully around the area, if at all.

Using all your fingers press up the calf, alternating your hands in firm, short pressing strokes. Stroke gently to the back of the knee and up the thigh right into the buttock. Repeat this move three times, starting just above the ankle and pressing the heel of your hands into the leg with the same alternate strokes.

Next, start at the buttock and work back down the leg, squeezing in a wringing, twisting motion. Upon reaching the ankle region wring up the leg and back down again.

Cover the left leg and move to the other leg. Repeat the steps for buttocks, hips, and legs on the right side. Remember to work rhythmically and apply more oil if you need it. Continue to check with the recipient to assess the quality of your touch.

The Halfway Point

You are now halfway through the massage and on your way to the next half, which is the front of the recipient's body. In transition to the next phase, adjust the cover so your recipient is completely draped. Standing at the side of the table, place your hands on the recipient's shoulders, with your fingers pressing in slightly. Lift your hands up a bit using the lift as leverage for your pressing fingers. Using steady rhythm, press in two lines down the body, on either side of the spine. Continue pressing over the buttocks and down the back of the legs. Press over the heels and down the length of the soles to the toes. Just below the ball of each foot, at the root of the toes, press your fingers in and hold for a count of three. With the same pressing rhythm, move back up the entire body to the shoulders, following the same two imaginary lines. Repeat your pressing movements, starting at the shoulders, working back down the body, ending in the center of the soles. Ⓔ

Chapter 7

Applying the Strokes: Front

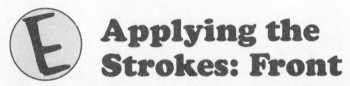

Don't let your session end with massaging the back of your partner's body without addressing the front. Remember that tension builds up throughout all the muscles. The muscles of the arms and upper chest are involved every time you lift, push, hold, or carry. The muscles in the front of the legs hold just as much tension as those in the back. Facial muscles also respond very well to massage. To complete your partner's relaxation it is essential that you massage the front as well as the back.

Turning Over

After you have massaged the back half of the receiver's body, he feels completely relaxed and is melting into the table. Although the idea of continuing sounds good, your massage partner probably would rather not move. Your request to turn over might be greeted with groans of resistance, so treat this time carefully. Speak quietly and offer assistance if it is needed. Always hold up the cover to ensure continued privacy while your receiver turns over.

FIGURE 7-1

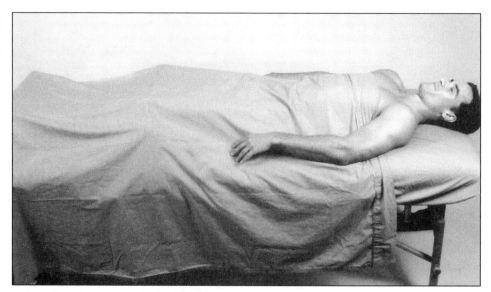

▲ Receiver is face up and covered.

Ask how the receiver feels as he rolls over. Suggest that the recipient be aware of the muscles you have just massaged, and check to see if turning over is easy or difficult. Ask if the recipient feels stiff or is able to move effortlessly. If the recipient feels stiffness, reassure him or her that sometimes the initial reaction to treating muscles is resistance. The reason is, you have just worked on a large group of muscles that may have been holding the body incorrectly, and you have changed the operation of these muscles, giving them a suggestion of how to work properly. Muscles have memory, so the old memory may try to assert itself, causing an achy feeling as the muscles work in a new way.

Continued massage will sustain the suggestion you have initiated. In addition, encourage the recipient to drink plenty of water throughout the day to flush out any toxins released through massage; these toxins can also cause muscles to feel achy after the toxins are released.

Once the recipient has turned over, settle the cover over his or her body as shown in **FIGURE 7-1**.

Check now to see where bolsters, pillows, or rolled towels are needed. If you were using a face cradle attached to the front of the table, remove it so you have easy access to that end of the table. Often folks like a pillow or two placed under their knees and calves to take pressure off their lower backs.

If the receiver can manage it, use nothing under the head, or just a small rolled towel behind the neck. You want easy access to the neck and upper back, and sometimes pillows get in the way. However, remember that the comfort of your recipient is primary; if your massage partner wants a pillow under the head, provide one. Let your receiver settle in, relaxing again as you check his or her comfort level once more.

Feet and Legs from the Front

Stand at the foot of the table, resting your hands on the tops of both feet. Breathe gently for a moment, feeling the heat from your hands spread out over the receiver. Undrape the left leg, tucking the cover between the two legs and folding the remaining length over the right leg. Support the left foot with your left hand, while the fingers of the right hand gently stroke down the top of the foot from ankle to toes. Smooth and press from the toes to the ankle; pull back up and press down again. Look at **FIGURE 7-2** to check your hand positions.

Now, let both hands rest with thumbs on top so that your hands are cupping the sole of the foot. With a steady circular motion make imaginary lines with your thumbs from the toes to the ankle and back to the toes. Cover the entire foot with these imaginary lines. Gently press your thumbs between bones, stimulating the tendons and muscles on the top surface of the foot.

FIGURE 7-2

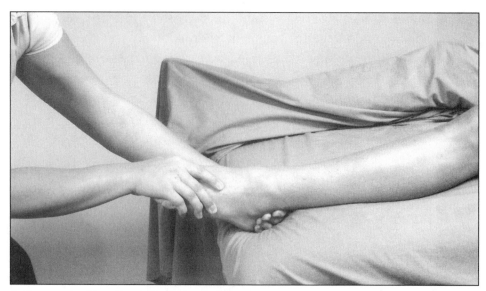

▲ Finger stroking the top of the foot.

Next, lower the foot to the table and place your hands on either side of the foot, gently shaking and rocking the foot side to side three times. Keeping your hands on either side of the foot, with the flat of your palms on the edges, rub the foot along the sides in a circular movement.

Shift the cover to the recipient's left leg and move to the right foot. Begin with your finger strokes at the ankle and repeat the same movements you performed on the left foot. Before you continue up the leg, cover the recipient's feet and wash your hands.

Moving Up the Front of the Legs

Place both your hands on the calf of the recipient's left leg, just above the ankle, and stroke up the leg with long smooth strokes as shown in **FIGURE 7-3**.

Your hands rest on the surface of the leg, pressing and stroking up to the hip. As you move up the leg, use firm steady pressure pressing toward the heart. Apply gliding strokes with a lighter touch as you work down to the ankle. Repeat this move three times, making sure you press and stroke around the entire hip. Move your body along the side of the leg as you stroke up and back.

Next, work your way up the entire leg, using the circular kneading technique as shown in **FIGURE 7-4**.

FIGURE 7-3

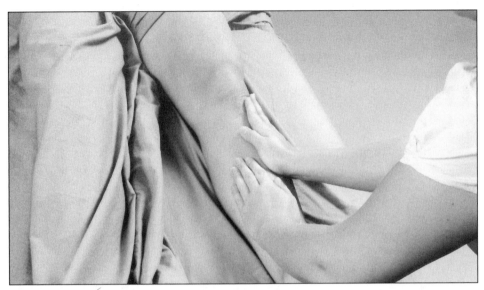

▲ Long gliding strokes from the ankle to the hip.

FIGURE 7-4

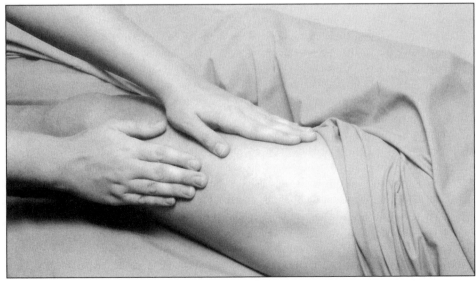

▲ Circular kneading up the front of the leg.

Use the pads of your fingers as you circle and pull the muscles along the shin and thigh. Lay your hands flat, then lift up to your fingers as you circle and press forward. Continue this circle-press-forward motion up the leg to the area around the hip. Move your fingers in toward the inner side of the hip bone and then circle out applying steady even pressure. Check with your receiver to make sure you are not pressing too hard.

Petrissage the Upper Leg

Stand on the right side to work on the outside of the recipient's left thigh. Reach across with both hands to lift and knead the thigh. **FIGURE 7-5** indicates where you should place your hands.

FIGURE 7-5

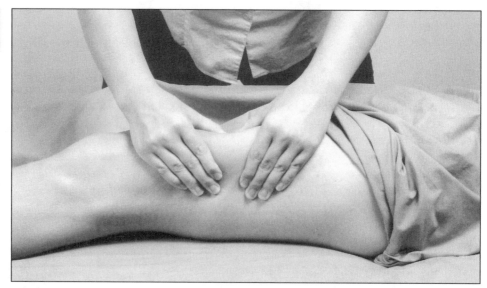

▲ Lift and knead the flesh of the thigh.

Hold the flesh of the thigh between your fingers while you knead along the entire outside of the upper leg. Return to just above the knee and repeat the movement up to the top of the leg, just below the cover. Knead and lift along the entire thigh surface using less pressure on the inside of the thigh.

Wring and Roll

Move to the left side of the recipient and grasp the left leg at the ankle with both hands. Your hands face the other leg with your palms resting on the outside of the leg and your fingers on the inside. Wring up the entire length of the leg and back down, repeating twice. Now place one hand under the leg and one on top and make a rolling motion. Your hands roll the leg as you roll up along the entire leg and back down. Do this at least twice.

Drape the left leg and move to the right leg. Tuck the cover from the right leg between the recipient's legs and let any excess drape over the left leg. Repeat all steps on the right leg, remembering to apply oil as needed.

Massaging the Abdomen

The abdomen is an area where you need to be especially conscious of your receiver's comfort. Some people love to have their bellies massaged while others do not. If your recipient doesn't want you to massage this area, proceed to the chest and arms.

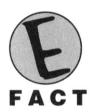

FACT

The abdomen contains the organs of digestion and elimination. Massage of the abdominal area supports the functions of these organs and improves circulation to the muscles in this part of the body.

If you decide to massage the abdomen, first drape the receiver properly, using a bath towel to cover the upper body of a female receiver. Tuck the larger cover around the hips. Stand to the right side of the body for easy hand placement, and begin circling with large gliding strokes from right to left three times, covering the entire abdomen. Look at **FIGURE 7-6** to see where your hands begin in this move.

FIGURE 7-6

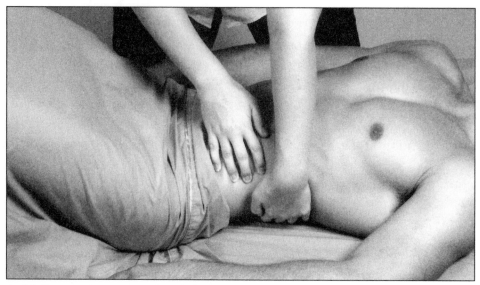

▲ Gliding strokes across the abdomen.

Next, knead this region from right to left three to five times. Then go back over the entire abdomen with small deep circles, pressing your fingers in deeply. Continue to massage again, using your entire hand to make deep gliding strokes, pulling across the abdomen in horizontal lines. Gently stretch the skin away from the center of the abdomen to the sides. Complete this part of the massage by resting your hands gently on the abdomen, allowing the heat from your hands to flow into the receiver. When finished, pull the large cover back up to the shoulders and gently remove the towel from under the drape.

The Chest and Front of the Arms

As you prepare to massage the upper body, make sure the cover is tucked in with the recipient's arms resting on top. Stand on the left side of the body and begin with the recipient's left arm. Apply oil with firm long strokes up and down the arm with one hand, as shown in **FIGURE 7-7**. Use your other hand to support the arm as the receiver relaxes, allowing you to take over.

FIGURE 7-7

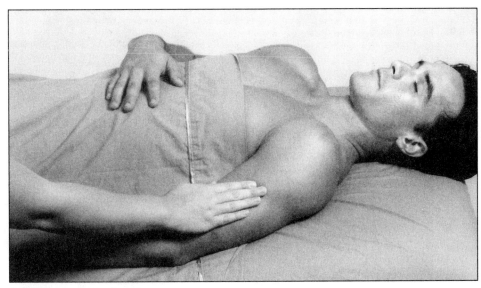

▲ Effleurage up the arm.

Bring both hands on top of the arm and wring the arm from the wrist to the shoulder and back again. Feel the arm relaxing as you wring back and forth three times.

Support the arm again while the palms and fingers of your working hand make deep circular strokes from the elbow up to the shoulder. Each time you reach the shoulder, feather down and off slightly. Finally, lift and knead the flesh of the arm from the wrist to the shoulder, actually picking up the skin and muscle. Most people find this feels exceptionally good, but check with your receiver to make sure the deep kneading friction is all right for him or her.

The Elbow

Hold one of your hands under the recipient's elbow and use the thumb and fingers of your other hand to work the small muscles of the elbow. Your thumb is on the inside of the elbow and your fingers are on the outside. Be very careful not to press too hard. Use small circular motions first with your thumb and then with your fingers as you can see in **FIGURE 7-8**.

FIGURE 7-8

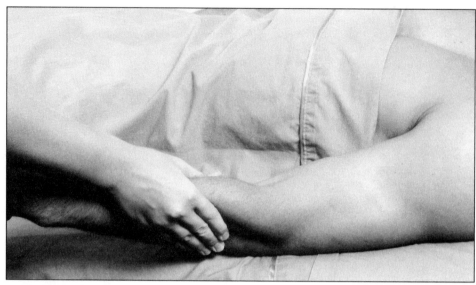

▲ Circle on the elbow.

Lastly, apply circle kneading around the entire elbow, including the bony areas. Use your fingers and work all around them. Do not press hard!

The Hands

Hold the recipient's left hand in your left hand and grasp one of the recipient's fingers with your right hand. Press your thumb down each finger as shown in **FIGURE 7-9**.

After you press with your thumb down each finger, use your thumb and index finger to press and roll between each finger on the muscular area between each finger. Turn the recipient's hand palm up and use both your thumbs to wring the palm. Wring up and down the hand three times before stretching across the palm with both your thumbs, also three times.

FIGURE 7-9

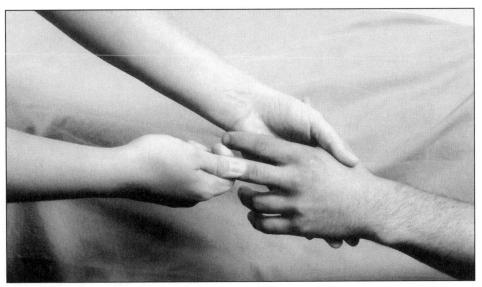

▲ Thumb press down on fingers.

The Shoulder

Still on the left side, use both your hands to glide up the recipient's arm to the shoulder. At the shoulder, circle the entire area on the top of the arm, using deep kneading strokes. Slide your left hand under the shoulder blade and continue to knead along the top of the shoulder to the neck with your right hand. Feel the muscles along the upper arm as you knead in deep circular motions.

Supporting with both your hands, extend the recipient's arm palm up, out from the side of the body and up toward the ear. Move the entire arm in circles. You can see what this range of motion movement looks like in **FIGURE 7-10**. Circle only as far as the arm is comfortable moving, so be sure to check with your receiver.

Repeat the massage on the right arm and shoulder before moving on to the chest.

FIGURE 7-10

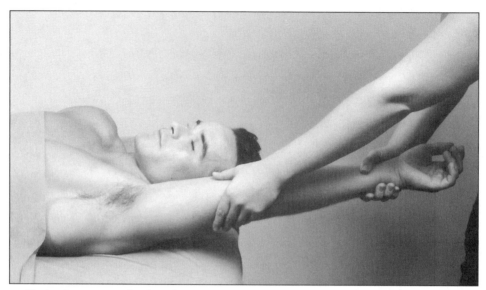

▲ Circle the arm at the head.

The Chest

Make sure the cover is securely tucked beneath the recipient's armpits, particularly for a female recipient. Then, stand at the head of your receiver, placing both your hands just below the neck on the top surface of the chest. The fingers of each hand touch each other and your palms are resting away from the center. Gently press down on this area, using very little pressure.

To continue on a male recipient, move to the side of the body, facing the receiver, and place your hands on one side of the chest. Use your fingers to gently circle across the chest with imaginary horizontal lines. The pressure should be steady but light. Repeat three times. After the last circle across, press both your hands on the upper chest surface and hold, to a count of five, then release.

Massaging the Back from the Front

Stand behind the recipient's head and to one side with your hands palm up. Gently slide both your hands under the left side of the back, with your fingers pressing into the back. As you move your arms down under the body, bend your knees so you have better control of your pressure and your body. In this bent-knee stance, stop when your arms can reach no further down the back. Keep the backs of your hands resting on the table and press your fingers slightly into the back. Slowly begin to move back toward your body, pressing your fingers and pulling your arms as you move.

Your fingers will feel any tightness or congested areas as you pull back. Stop on an area of congestion and move your fingers in small circular motions, still pressing in with your fingers. Circle on an area three times and continue to pull back, eventually straightening your body as you pull your arms out from under the back. Go in again and repeat this stroke before moving to the other side where you will apply the same technique.

The Neck

To massage the neck, begin by oiling along the top of the shoulders and up along the sides and back of the neck. Turn the head to one side as you gently stroke oil on the neck with one hand and hold the head with your other. Turn the head to the other side and glide oil on this side of the neck, again holding the head with your other hand. Turn the head forward and cradle the neck in both hands, exactly as in **FIGURE 7-11**. Your fingers are pressing in under the neck and your thumbs are at the sides of the neck.

Using circular motions press your fingers in and gently circle and knead the back of the neck. This is another area to treat with extreme sensitivity, so check with your receiver to see if he is still comfortable.

Now, turn the head to one side, using one hand to support the head, and circle along the side of the neck with the fingers of your other hand. Move from the top of the shoulders into the neck, kneading the entire area. Press your fingers in along the neck, working up to the occipital ridge (the bony ridge under the ear). Refer to **FIGURE 7-12** for proper hand position.

At the occipital ridge press and hold to a count of five. Repeat this stroke three times. Then turn the head to the other side and repeat your circling and kneading on this side of the neck.

FIGURE 7-11

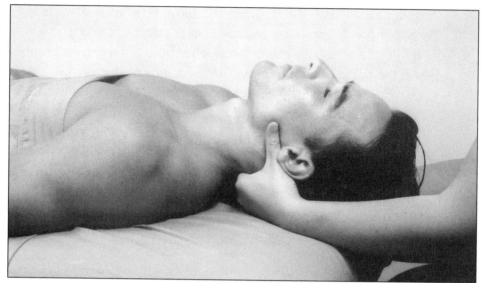

▲ The head rests in your hands.

FIGURE 7-12

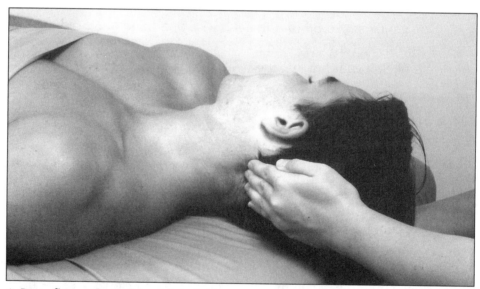

▲ Press fingers in at the occipital ridge.

Now, cup both hands under the back of the neck. With the head flat on the table, gently pull the head. Hold for three counts and release, pressing your hands down and gliding along the tops of the shoulders. Repeat twice.

Working the Face, Head, and Scalp

Stand at the end of the table and begin the face massage with both hands on the recipient's chin. Apply a pinching motion with your thumbs and index fingers from the center of the chin to the edge of the jaw and back. Repeat at least three times. Use the fingers of both hands and walk from the chin to under the mouth. Use your thumbs to walk with a creeping motion in lines from the jaw over the cheeks to the sides of the face. Use either your thumb or fingers to walk from the jaw between the mouth and nose.

Starting at the sides of the face along the jaw, use your thumbs and index fingers of both hands to pinch and roll as you knead up both cheeks. This is a wonderful technique for sagging, tired skin. As you knead up the sides of the face the receiver will feel the blood returning to the skin tissue. In the same upward direction, use a circling friction motion with your fingers to further stimulate the muscles of the face.

Use circular strokes on the forehead with your thumbs, as in **FIGURE 7-13**.

FIGURE 7-13

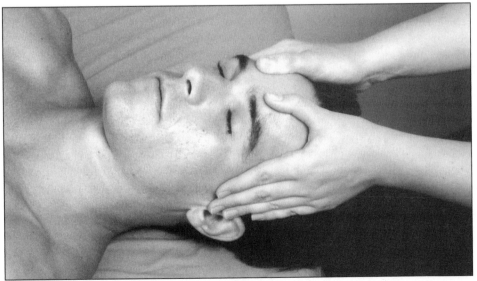

▲ Circular motion of thumbs on the forehead.

As you finish the thumb circles on the forehead, stroke the entire face with both hands from the jaw up to the top of the forehead. Bring your hands right on to the scalp and, using your finger pads, circle the top and sides of the head.

Rest your hands gently on the top of the head and feel the heat of your hands penetrate the receiver.

Quiet Touch

All good things come to an end, and finishing with your receiver's head is the end of your full-body massage, at least for now. But before it is ended today, close your session with a quiet, peaceful energy, which will allow the receiver to transition easily to the reality of his or her outside life.

Stand at the head of your recipient, gently placing your hands on the shoulders. Breathe easily and quietly, transmitting a sense of peace and calm to the receiver. Press in gently yet firmly with your hands and hold. Feel the shoulders relax further as the body sinks into the table.

Very gently and smoothly stroke down the arms and legs, right through the cover. The idea here is to tuck in the good feeling, instilling a sense of quiet wholeness to your receiver. Move down to the feet, gently resting your hands here. Again breathe slowly and evenly as you quietly rest at the feet.

The experience of massage will last long after the receiver comes off the table. The energy of the environment you have created along with the relaxing service you have provided will remain for some time. Leave the recipient as you go wash your hands, allowing for a few moments of complete quiet. If you can give the receiver three to five minutes of undisturbed rest, how grand!

When you return, let the receiver know he should get up slowly, enjoying the moments of calmness. Ask if your help is needed, and if it is not, give the receiver privacy to dress and come out of the room. Offer water and ask the recipient to sit for a moment.

You have completed your first massage with many more to come. The wonder of massage is that you can repeat this over and over again. But remember, receiving is as good as giving, so make sure you have someone who will practice on *you*.

Chapter 8

Understanding and Relieving Stress

Stress is a function of life; without it you do not exist. How you react to stress dictates whether or not you are distressed. Distress becomes disease, so the key to stress is leaning how to deal with the forces of life with ease. To flow through life without effort, embracing every situation as a lesson and using the tools you discover, is a goal worth achieving. Massage is a tool that can help you learn to go with the flow.

Stress Is the Life Force

To be alive is to have stress. The challenges that stress presents provide the stimulus we all need to live. Without the motivation of stress we would not think and we certainly would not act. The rhythm of life flows from the essence that is stress.

Your reaction to stress is the way you respond to an event, or stressor. Typically people view stressors as threats to their peace and well-being, resulting in a reaction. Stressors generally cause people to worry, feel overloaded, respond with anger, or become depressed. The result is that they feel they must protect themselves from any real or perceived event, particularly if the event is out of their control. Does this sound familiar to you?

Daily Stress

Every activity you do involves stress because stress is part of living. Your positive response to stress allows you to survive with gusto, taking in all that life has to offer. Your daily routine consists of activities you have adapted to—your body, mind, and emotions generally know what to expect and they become comfortable with the routine. So the stress of your day-to-day life flows fairly well, but suddenly—zap—something happens to change your routine, and that disruption becomes a stressor.

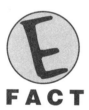

FACT

Any change, even a pleasant one, can cause stress. Changing jobs or going on vacation is a stress. However, a change that you control affects you in a different way from a change you don't control. If you lose your job or cannot afford a vacation, you will experience that stress much differently from the stress you feel looking forward to a new job or a fun getaway.

Too much stress, even of your own choosing, can cause havoc. If you thrive on chaos and constant upheaval, eventually your lifestyle will catch up with you. Assuming too much responsibility, creating undue pressure, thriving on overstimulation will cause an eventual imbalance. One of the biggest challenges facing people today is how to achieve a state of balance when dealing with stress.

Recharge Your Body

The flight from danger or the need to fight for food does not exist on such a primal level today. However, a stressful meeting or an emotional confrontation still creates a highly charged physical response in us. Our body's reaction is normal, because, unfortunately, evolution has not caught up with our need to adapt our fight-or-flight response to present-day realities. Therefore, we often stay at a highly charged level, with our bodies running on high, because physically fleeing or fighting doesn't often solve our problems today. After a fight-or-flight response to stress, our bodies need physical exercise to burn off excess energy, and then our bodies need rest to replenish our energy. Massage is one of the tools to help the body release stress, recharge the body, and renew the feeling of well-being.

Distress and Disease

The mechanisms of the body are constantly working to deal with the daily stresses of living. Homeostasis (the process of keeping the body in balance) keeps the internal functions of the body within normal levels as all the body systems work together in rhythm. If, however, stress goes beyond the normal limits, certain changes are triggered within the body. The physical response to stress is created by a chain reaction involving the central nervous system, the brain, and the production of certain hormones that explode through the bloodstream in the fight-or-flight reaction.

Stress has always been here from the inception of humankind, and we have responded to the threat of danger in exactly the same way throughout our history. The fact that the human race can deal with stress has guaranteed our survival. Ancient humans were able to react properly due to the actual physiological response that stressors produce, and the fight-or-flight response saved their lives. If an animal attacked them or they encountered a natural catastrophe, the response from within their bodies determined their survival. As you exist today, you are designed with a built-in lifesaver that gives you the extra strength you need to either stand and fight or run away with a tremendous burst of speed.

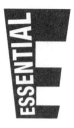

Think of the stories of mothers lifting cars off their fallen babies or of untrained civilians rescuing people from peril. The excessive rush of strength we get in the face of danger is due to the powerful way our bodies react to stressful or threatening situations.

The tales of unsung heroes, professional and accidental, illustrate the body's response to stress—the fast heartbeat, the elevated blood pressure, faster breathing, and an increase in muscle tension. The body is also designed to relax and de-stress after every incident of the fight-or-flight reaction. However, many people do not take the time or do not recognize the physiological and psychological need to wind down.

How the Mind Influences the Body

The connection between body and mind has long been established. Your thoughts influence your emotions, and your emotions influence your body, and a cycle of body, mind, and spirit evolves. Thinking is good, unless you obsess. Obsessive thinking becomes obsessive worrying and this results in ill health. To be healthy, you can help yourself by recognizing that you can reverse the way you respond to stress. By relaxing your body and your mind you can control your reactions as well as change how you deal with stressors.

Your mind can make you sick, but your mind can also help you stay well. As you become aware of the effects of stress, you can learn how to redirect your thoughts and emotions to create an atmosphere that supports good health. You have the ability to create a healthy environment for yourself by learning to change the way you think. Your brain affects your entire being, so relax your brain and you will relax your body.

The brain acts like the processor in your computer; it is the center of all ingoing and outgoing information. Every thought, feeling, sense, and function is controlled through the brain from messages carried back and forth via the spinal cord. Stress affects the operation of the brain directly through the hypothalamus and indirectly through the responses radiating from the body. You can help the brain function at its highest level by learning to relax. As the body learns to relax the mind can also relax, stilling the senses and rejuvenating the body. The power of your mind can keep you healthy and your body can help your mind to accomplish this task.

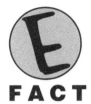

FACT

Deep relaxation of the brain produces homeostasis. As you relax, the body produces more chemicals that promote feelings of well-being, such as serotonin for mood control, dopamine for emotional response, and norepinephrine for dreaming. When these chemicals flow freely, all body systems function at their best and tension is released.

The Effects of Stress on the Body

Today's society is fast paced with the emphasis on fast and busy. Everyone seems to be in a huge hurry to do more, be more, and get more, and part of the way to achieve all this is to stay in a state of constant "up." The response of the body to stress is to become more—to think clearer, to function faster, to be stronger—all of this and not feel hungry! Many people are so used to operating at a high stress level that they do not want to come down. The initial feeling of sharp intelligence, quick wit, and tremendous endurance is exhilarating. For many the thought of not performing at this seemingly peak level is not conceivable. It is unfortunate that most people still do not realize the depleting demands of stress. For many the long-term effects of constant stress result in chronic illness.

Digestion and Elimination

Long-term stress can result in a number of health issues. Stress can be held in any organ or muscle of the body, so if you have an area of weakness, that area becomes a target for stress. Your stomach for one cannot keep on stomaching stress without damage! Ulcers and other digestive disorders are clearly linked to stress. Many people experience low-grade stomach upset every day and attribute this condition to a nervous stomach. If your stomach is nervous you have long-term stress.

Furthermore, many intestinal issues such as irritable bowel syndrome, inflammatory bowel, or colitis are aggravated by stress. The body's instinctive response to stress is to shut down the digestive and elimination functions; therefore chronic stress becomes a serious issue.

Stress and the Skin

One of the first places extended stress can be seen is in the skin. Your skin is visible and you can see how you look whenever you want— that can be a stress in itself on a day that your skin breaks out! The chemical imbalances caused by stress can change the condition of your skin, your hair, and your nails. All can become dry and dull, reflecting the effects of stress for all to see. Dry skin and dandruff as well as thin and cracked nails can also be a result of chronic stress. More severe skin conditions like acne, eczema, psoriasis, and even hives may come from stress.

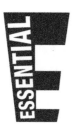

The human function curve is a concept developed by Dr. Peter Nixon, a cardiologist in London, to demonstrate the effects of long-term stress. Nixon showed that, initially, performance increases under stress; however, over the long term, fatigue introduces decline in performance and, finally, ill health and breakdown. He also showed that long-term stress produces unawareness of the performer as he or she begins to decline.

Your Heart and Your Lungs

Stress and the long-term effects of stress affect your blood pressure and the rate of your heartbeat. Constant stress on the heart muscle weakens its function. A weakened heart leads to a weakened circulatory system, which adds pressure on the lungs as well. If the lungs weaken, they are unable to bring enough oxygen into the body, which leads to the problem of how to release toxic waste. You can see how not dealing with stress creates a mess of the whole body.

Stress and Your Muscles

The tension that stress creates as it prepares you to fight or flee puts an incredible amount of pressure on your muscles. During times of great stress you are strong enough to defend yourself and also able to run unbelievably fast—more so than you normally would be. However, a prolonged stay in this condition may lead to a weakening of these muscles, and that can take away your overall strength and endurance. With the weakening of the muscles comes pain, and chronic pain is debilitating.

Imagine a condition where you try to use your body—walk, play with your child, take the trash out—and a tremendous pain runs through your hip, stopping you in your tracks. You drink some water and try again only to be hit with even more pain. You attempt to continue but your body will not let you. The next day you are fine, and you continue with your routine, only to be hit again a few days later, this time far worse than before.

To add insult to injury that night you can't sleep because of the pain. You take a few aspirins and hop into the shower, only to discover that now you hurt all over; even your skin hurts as the water hits it. This episode sends you to the doctor, who may or may not be aware of the painful intensity or encompassing scope of chronic pain syndrome. Let's hope your doctor is, because this pain is real; it is not in your head! People who suffer from burnout may experience this kind of pain, another side effect of stress.

Balance and Stress

The nervous system supports the immune system and the immune system supports balance in your body. Both of these systems work with the endocrine system to help keep your body and mind fine-tuned and in a constant state of homeostasis. Normal day-to-day living creates stress that these systems can deal with; however, a continued barrage of stress-related incidents that leave your head spinning affects the way your body fights off disease.

Keeping the mind, body, and spirit strong gives support to all the functions of the body. Massage and other forms of relaxation not only teach you to relax but strengthen your ability to stay healthy.

Release Through Massage

You want to reduce your stress, let go of your tension, and feel relaxed all at the same time. Massage provides all of this, allowing you to be in the moment with your body and free of any stressors. Massage heals and invigorates simultaneously. The different strokes are designed to enhance health while preventing an unhealthy response to stress.

Massage teaches you to relax, encouraging all the systems to be in balance. The manipulation of muscles and connective tissue releases congestion and helps to tone the body. The release of tension promotes physical well-being while removing memory of injury from the muscle. When you have a massage you are giving the muscles a positive experience, which helps you feel good both mentally and physically.

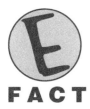

FACT

Muscle memory is the concept that states that muscles remember what the mind has taught. This is why it is difficult to change a poor habit such as slumping posture or holding your head at a tilt. When you hold yourself correctly, it will feel wrong because your muscles remember the old way.

The effects of massage deal with the body's stress response and promote a relaxation reaction. Massage improves circulation and lowers high blood pressure, which supports the heart. It helps with digestion, keeping that system functioning smoothly, too. The lymphatic system responds to massage by releasing toxins that could lead to illness. Massage also encourages the immune system. In addition, it triggers the production and release of endorphins, the feel-good hormones. Just as important, compassionate touch speaks to the human need for good, caring touch. Regular massage is an essential tool, teaching people how to react to stress with a healthy and relaxed response. By relaxing the muscles, you release tension, which helps you to face many situations with inner strength and a new outlook.

Other Relaxation Techniques

There are many relaxation techniques, in addition to massage, that provide you with the tools to relax and rejuvenate. Each one helps to combat the adverse effects of prolonged stress, prevent illness, and promote health. These techniques recognize the person as a whole being: body, mind, emotions, and soul. A person's emotional well-being is directly connected with physical health, and both are connected with the mind. There are a wide variety of ways that you can learn to manage your stress. It is a good idea to study a few and find what works for you. The following relaxation techniques can all be used in combination with a massage program to help maximize your own stress reduction.

Space Management

The practice of feng shui, the Chinese tradition of configuring space to harmonize with the spiritual forces that inhabit it, suggests that you should rid yourself of clutter. Whether you know it or not, clutter causes stress. So, if you have old magazines, puzzles, videos, eight-track tapes, clothes, and other possessions that you don't need, don't want, and keep thinking you might use one day, get rid of them! Have a yard sale or give your old good stuff to the Salvation Army, St. Vincent De Paul, or any other such nonprofit agency. Whatever you have been holding on to, thinking you will fix it someday, toss it out.

Once you begin to clear out, check in with yourself and see how you feel—great, right? Getting rid of stuff helps you get rid of stuff. Translation: If you clear out old things physically, you will clear out old things emotionally and mentally as well. Keep up the good work and happy clearing.

Aromatherapy

The smell of oranges—ahhh—reminds us of summer days with our families, or some other terrific memory. Some smells make us feel happy and some make us feel sad, while some release stress. Both aromatherapy and herbal teas have stress-releasing properties—the essential oils often come from certain herbs that make healing teas.

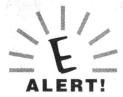

ALERT!

If you are pregnant, have a medical condition, or a tendency toward allergic reactions, check with your medical practitioner as well as a clinical aromatherapist and a trained herbalist before you use any oils or herbs. Never take essential oils internally.

Chamomile, which can be used in aromatherapy and as a tea, is an herb that reduces stress and promotes sleep. Rosemary, another herb that stimulates the nervous system, is produced as an oil for aromatherapy and as a tea. You will learn more about aromatherapy in Chapter 19.

Proper Nutrition

You are what you eat, and if you eat foods with high fat and low nutrition you are stressing your body. Today it seems as though everyone is involved in one fad diet or another, putting unnecessary stress on his or her body. Before you begin an eating plan, make sure that is exactly what you are doing—undertaking a *plan* that can become a lifestyle, not just starting a diet. There are organizations and numerous books on good nutrition that can offer you some basic guidelines so you can devise your own nutritionally sound style of eating.

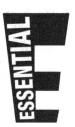

Junk food may taste good to some people, but it gives a rush of energy followed by a resounding crash. To reclaim that energetic feeling, many junk food eaters continue to eat those foods, which are deficient in nutrients, and end up starving their bodies.

Eating can be fun as well as sensible. Create a lifestyle full of fresh fruits and vegetables as well as salads. Pick foods for the vibrant colors they possess and arrange the food artistically. Choose organic foods, which are foods that are not treated with chemicals and hormones, substances that add to the stress level in your body. Organic grains, fish, meats, and poultry can help you to sustain a healthy body and mind.

Meditation

The principal concept of meditation is to release stress from your body by calming the central nervous system. As the central nervous system becomes calm, you learn to stay in the present moment, to be still with yourself in body, mind, and spirit. Meditation calms the body and the mind so that you can resolve the issues that cause you stress, be they anger, depression, pain, or fear.

There are many forms of meditation and just as many books to tell you how to meditate. Try to find one that fits for you. A good place to start is with prayer, one of the oldest forms of meditation and positive affirmation. Use prayers that are familiar to you and set aside a particular time of day to practice. The longer you practice, the calmer and happier you will feel.

You may move on from your familiar prayers to other meditations or stay with what you know; the important issue is to find what works for you and practice. Even with a busy schedule, you can set aside five to ten minutes a day to calm your mind. Try early in the morning before you start your day or before you go to bed as the last part of your nighttime routine, whatever works. Be disciplined and you will benefit.

Exercise

Exercise helps to decrease the effects of stress in a number of ways. Exercise builds muscle, improves your circulation, and rids your body of congestion caused by toxins. Exercise helps you to deal with stress because it encourages your nervous and endocrine systems to produce the chemicals that counteract stress. Remember the fight-or-flight stress response? Exercise replicates the fighting/fleeing and tells your body that you have done your job and that your body can return to normal. As you finish exercising, your body recognizes that the danger is over and the relaxation phase can begin.

The key to sticking with an exercise program is finding one that fits your lifestyle. If you like being at home, pick something that you can do without leaving the house, like yoga or Pilates. Even tai chi can be done in the privacy of your home. Of course, there are plenty of exercise classes, too, if you prefer a group. A gym offers many options and most gyms have classes in many different types of exercise as well as personal trainers and massage therapists. And don't forget walking, which is free.

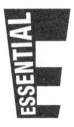

The deal with stress management and relaxation techniques is that you have to make a commitment to follow through, which means you have to enjoy the technique. Find one (or many) that resonate with you. If you don't like what you find here, fine; design your own technique—take what you do like and devise something that works for you.

Once you make a choice, try working with a program for one month before deciding either you love it or you want to try something different. Whatever you choose, be it one form or many, have fun and take a friend.

Bodywork

Massage is only one of many types of bodywork to choose from, and any form of bodywork is a de-stressor. See Chapter 18 to read more about reflexology, Reiki, lomilomi, and other forms of bodywork and specialized massage techniques. Within the range of choices you will find something to your liking. The chief issue to consider when choosing bodywork is what exactly appeals to you, because that will dictate what you are willing to try.

Massage is a stress management tool that creates a healthy reaction to life. The very act of relaxing enough to receive a massage begins the act of releasing stress, and massage in itself can be a form of meditation. Caring and compassionate touch supports the mind, body, and spirit connection, creating an environment that is healthy and sympathetic. The joy of living replaces the strain of stress as you utilize some of the tools you have discovered. Enjoy every moment of being. Ⓔ

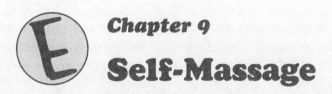

Chapter 9

Self-Massage

Massage is a wonderful gift for everyone, including you, the giver. To be a good massage practitioner you need to know what the receiver feels. Practicing the massage techniques on yourself gives you an understanding of how you feel to others. Performing the strokes first on yourself lets you experiment in a way that is beneficial, because you can experience the effects of your touch and critique your own work. Self-massage is a relaxing experience. Try it—you will like it!

Stretching and Breathing

The beauty of self-massage is you can do it anywhere. You can be clothed or not, sitting, standing, or lying down. Begin with a stretch by clasping your fingers together as you stretch your arms out in front, palms facing each other, opening up your shoulders. Unclasp your hands and stretch your arms overhead, palms facing, as you gently rotate your head side to side. Stretch your torso from one side to the other, still reaching with your arms. Lastly, gently stretch your arms to the side, holding them out from your shoulders with your palms up. Let your arms come down to the sides of your body; you are ready to begin.

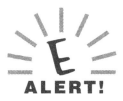

ALERT!

Know your body's limitations. When performing any stretching exercise do not overdo! Stretch in each direction within the framework of your own body. Adapt each maneuver, recognizing and embracing your comfort zone. Always listen to every signal your body sends you.

Rest both hands on your stomach area, one above the belly button and one below. Close your eyes for a moment and breathe. Feel your lungs expand and contract and notice that your diaphragm is moving right below your rib cage. As you inhale your abdomen expands and your belly pushes up. When you exhale your belly contracts, helping to push the air up and out of your body. As your hands rise and fall with each breath celebrate the cleansing your body is experiencing.

An Exercise in Silence

To be silent is a gift you may give to yourself. To begin pick a time when you know you will not be interrupted. Perhaps this means getting up fifteen minutes earlier than others in your household, or staying up fifteen minutes later. Maybe you work at home and you can take fifteen minutes to be alone sometime during your workday. If you are parenting a newborn or toddler, plan your silent time during baby's naptime.

Cover yourself with a light blanket and sit or lie quietly, with your eyes closed and your palms face up. Breathe in slowly and fully, letting your breath fill your abdomen. Release your breath completely and continue to follow this pattern with slow, quiet breathing. Listen to your body as your heartbeat begins to speak, bringing your awareness to the rhythm of your pulses. Relax into this rhythm, letting go of any connection outside your body.

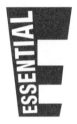

Many people feel that it is selfish to set aside personal time. Selfishness means not sharing the gifts of your abundance, like not sharing extra food or clothing. It is not selfish to feed yourself first; if you are not sustained, you cannot sustain anyone else.

Visualize yourself sitting or lying in a huge tub, relaxed, ready to receive. Picture someone you love approaching with a huge pitcher filled with a golden liquid; the word "love" is floating on top of the fluid. As you rest, your partner pours endless amounts of golden love over you, washing you completely, allowing you to feel full of love. Relax and allow this feeling to flow through your body. Become aware of your breathing again and slowly stretch and open your eyes.

Massaging Your Abdomen

The abdomen is the center of your being. Many important organs are housed within this area of your body. Some cultures feel that the abdomen is the seat of the soul. In many traditional eastern philosophies the abdomen is known as the hara, the center of the life force.

Touching the center of yourself is to honor you. You don't have to take off your clothes; just sit or lie in a comfortable space. Whether you use oil for this exercise will depend upon your state of dress or undress. You can perform all the strokes without oil if you prefer. Place your hands gently on your abdomen, and feel the light touch. Relax as your hands press lightly on your body, creating a moment of quiet release. This is the holding stroke.

Rest one hand on your thigh while the other hand glides in a circle around your abdomen. Always start on your right side and move clockwise. The large intestine (the colon) begins just above your pubic bone on the right side of your body. It curves up the right side, across the waist to the left, and then down along the left side before reaching the rectum. Massage strokes support the function of the inner organs; therefore you work in the direction of movement. The colon is the last stop before excretion of solids from the body, so you massage in the direction of elimination. The gliding strokes support the process of movement, freeing toxins and relaxing the colon.

Surface kneading of the abdomen allows the blood to circulate, toning the skin. Using both hands, grasp the skin of your abdomen between your fingers and thumbs, lift up, pinch, and roll. Knead with both hands, moving from below your belly up to your ribs and then down again. Bring your hands to the sides of your abdomen and knead in toward the center with the pinching, rolling motion. When your fingers meet, stretch and roll the skin back to your sides.

Bring both hands to the lower right section of your abdomen and knead deeply, using your fingers to press in before you lift, pinch, and roll. Move up along the right side to your rib cage, following the path of the ascending colon. Continue the motion across your waistline and down the left side, turning in toward the lower center of your abdomen. Work with this press-lift-pinch-roll rhythm over your entire abdominal surface.

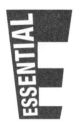

Working on the abdominopelvic region will release pockets of toxins from the small and large intestines. Belching and flatulence caused by excessive amounts of air in the stomach or intestines may accompany the release of toxins. Your body is a wonderful creation equipped with many tools that aid in proper function. The body's ability to release gas is one of these tools.

Bring your hands to the sides of your body, just above your hipbones. Lift, pinch, and roll the flesh here, kneading up and down the sides of your abdomen. Complete the massage of your abdominal area by gently circling the entire area with clockwise strokes.

Shoulders, Arms, and Hands

Remain in a comfortable seated or lying position and move your hands from your abdomen up to your shoulders, lightly resting your hands on them, then gliding down and off. Repeat this gliding stroke across your shoulders three or four times. Stroke the top and back of your shoulders as though you are throwing away any burdens you may be carrying.

Using one hand on the opposite shoulder, start where your shoulder meets your neck, and knead your shoulder between your fingers and thumbs, or between your fingers and the heel of your palm. As you can see in **FIGURE 9-1**, your fingers work on the back of your shoulder while your thumb or heel of your palm works on the inside.

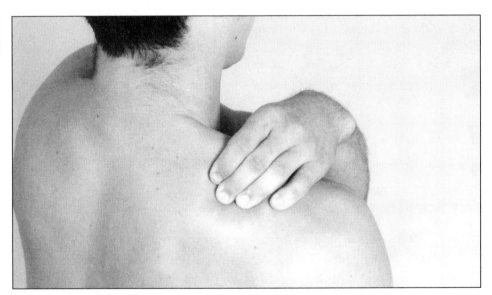

▲ Kneading stroke on the shoulder.

Grasp the skin and muscle along the line of your shoulder, moving out to the edge. Repeat this at least three times on each shoulder.

Now using both hands, place your fingers on both shoulders to press and stroke off. This movement is the same throwaway movement you used to start your shoulder massage but this time your fingers stroke in a different style. Let your fingers press into the back of your shoulders first and then pull off. Move up from the broad part of your shoulders to your upper shoulder while you press and pull. "Listen" with your fingers to identify any tight areas. If you find tightness, use a friction stroke with small deep circles and narrow in on the troublesome areas. Circle and press until you feel the tightness loosening. Using the same friction stroke on one shoulder at a time, push with your fingertips down the ridge of your shoulder and onto the top of the back. Press and glide, press and glide along your shoulder to the top of your arm, feeling the tight areas under your fingertips. Repeat. Then move to your other shoulder and press and stroke off, trying to find any tight areas in that shoulder, too.

With both hands on either side of your neck, brush lightly down from the curve in your neck to the top of your arms, sealing the work you have just performed. Brush with your hands three or four times. Raise your hands up off your shoulders and repeat these strokes. The brushing movements are meant to brush your aura.

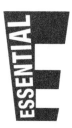

Your aura is part of your energy field—the space just outside your body that is invisible yet measurable. The aura has seven layers, each with its own function. These layers coincide with the seven major chakras, or wheels of energy. The seven layers deal with your physical, emotional, and spiritual development.

Moving Down the Arms

Start with one arm outstretched and the opposite hand resting on the top of your outstretched hand. Breathe and begin. Glide your open top hand up your arm to your shoulder and back to your hand several times. Feel your skin and underlying muscles relax with the gentle stroking as you glide over the entire surface of your arm. Grasp your arm between your fingers and your thumb, your fingers on the top side with your thumb on the bottom side, and rub up your arm using a friction stroke. Your skin will feel hot and tingly as your blood circulates to the surface of your arm. Repeat on your other arm.

Now begin kneading your upper arm, starting at the top of your elbow and working up to the shoulder. Using firm, grasping strokes, knead the muscles in the front of your arm and then knead the muscles on the back of your arm. Knead up to your shoulder. Then glide back down your arm, and knead up again, covering the entire surface of your upper arm. Make sure to work the underside of your upper arm right into your underarm area. Massage your underarm area using small circular strokes and round gliding strokes. Repeat on your other arm.

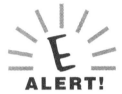

ALERT!

Because it has soft skin and many lymph nodes, the underarm area is quite sensitive, requiring you to work very slowly and gently. The upper inner arm along the length of the bone must be worked firmly but also gently because this area contains many nerve passageways.

Now work your forearm using the thumb and index finger of your opposite hand, lifting and pinching the skin from your wrist to your elbow, covering your entire forearm. Move from your wrist up to your elbow in a straight line, then glide down to your wrist and work up again in another line. Do this stroke over your entire forearm. Repeat the up-and-down kneading, but this time use all your fingers (not just your index finger) in a grasping, kneading motion, as you can see in **FIGURE 9-2**. Your forearm will feel energized.

FIGURE 9-2

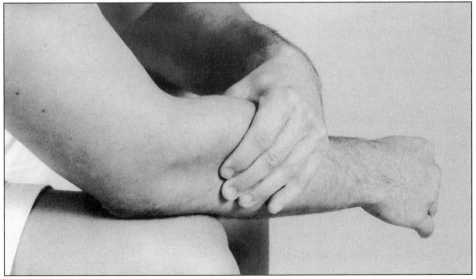

▲ Kneading stroke on the forearm.

Make sure you work all around your elbow with kneading and circling strokes. The muscles and tendons in this area are often tight from repetitive motion. Working in the elbow area relieves congestion and stress not only at the elbow but in the entire arm. Move to your other arm and massage in the same way, starting with the lifting and pressing strokes at your wrist.

Massaging the Hands

Wring your hands together, consciously feeling every part of your hands. Clap your hands together until they tingle. Tap your fingertips and thumbs at least ten times; then press and hold to the count of ten. Extend your arms, turn them slightly so the backs of your hands meet, and clap. Wring one wrist and then the other at least five times.

Next, press your index finger into the web between the thumb and index finger of your opposite hand, and hold the other side of the web with your thumb. Using a slight rolling motion, press along from the bottom of the web up to the top, holding your hands in the position shown in **FIGURE 9-3**. Repeat on the other hand.

FIGURE 9-3

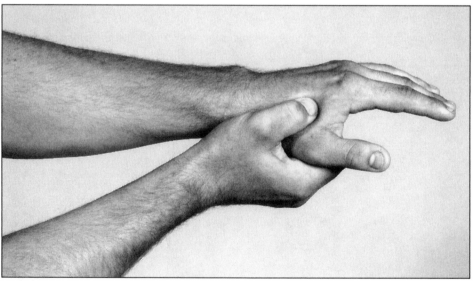

▲ Rolling stroke in the web of the thumb.

Finally, knead your closed fist into your open palm; then use your fingers to press and circle over your entire open palm. Switch hands and repeat these strokes. Finish by gliding off both palms with soft stroking movements, letting each hand stroke the other as if you are wiping off your hands.

Massaging Your Lower Body

By lower body, we mean hips, legs, and feet. The hips attach to the legs and provide support for them; the thigh bones, shinbones, and ultimately the feet carry the weight of the body. The feet support and balance the body when you walk or stand. It is obvious that these areas get quite a workout and can carry as much tension as your upper body.

Your Hips

Standing with both hands on your hips, circle in a gliding effleurage movement, warming up the area. With your fingertips on both hips make small deep circles along the hips and buttocks. Cover the entire area and repeat. Now, using your fingers and thumbs lift, pinch, and roll over your hips and buttocks, paying attention to any painful or tight areas. Focus on those areas with your finger pads, pressing and circling each point, then holding for a count of three. Move to each spot at least twice. After this movement, knead again with your fingers and thumbs over the entire hip and buttock area. To finish, circle and glide over the hips and buttocks, covering the area completely.

Upper Leg: Your Thigh

Sit now as you glide both your hands along one thigh from your hip to your knee and back up again in long circular motions over the front, sides, and back. Next, grasp the flesh and knead up and down your entire thigh, from hip to knee, in an imaginary line along the front, back, and sides. Again, feel for areas of sensitivity, and work deeper in tight areas while using less pressure in areas that are too painful. Repeat on your other thigh.

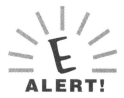

ALERT!

Use caution in the upper thigh and groin area, where the front part of the leg touches the torso. This area is a major pathway for veins and arteries. Too much pressure can cut off circulation. Behind the knee is another area sensitive to pressure, so massage there lightly as well.

With one hand on the outer thigh of each leg, follow the bones down the sides using circular pressure strokes. When you reach the outer edge of your knees circle around the tops of the kneecaps and work up your inner thighs. At the top of your thighs, circle and press down the center of your thighs to your knees again. Circle along the tops of your knees to the outside of your thighs; then circle and press up the bones to your hips, where you press and hold for a count of three. Repeat this pattern three times.

Massaging one leg at a time, move your hand to the back of your thigh (use the hand on the same side as the thigh you are working). Working from just under your buttock, circle and press down the back of your thigh to the soft tissue behind your knee. Gently stroke the area behind your knee, but do not circle or press. Work back up your thigh, continuing to circle and press imaginary vertical lines from your buttock to the back of your knee, up and down the back of your thigh, until you reach the inner side of your thigh.

Using your other hand, press and knead the same thigh in small horizontal lines back and forth across the inner side of your thigh, up to the outer side of your buttock. Then glide over the entire thigh front to back, using deep pressure for two complete gliding strokes. Begin to change the pressure on the third stroke and glide lightly over your upper thigh a few more times for closure. Repeat on the other thigh.

Lower Leg: Your Calf and Shin

To work your calf, either sit down and cross your leg over the opposite thigh, or stand and rest your foot on a stool. Using both hands glide over your calf first. Then use both hands to knead the back of your calf from the ankle to the knee as shown in **FIGURE 9-4**.

FIGURE 9-4

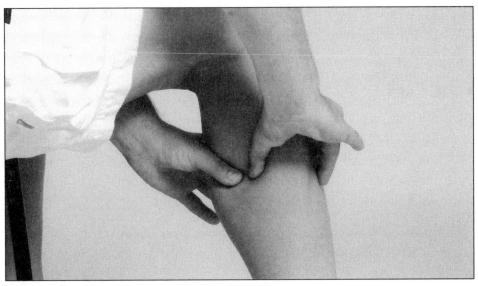

▲ Kneading stroke up the calf.

As you focus on the center of the calf you may actually feel the two separate parts of the muscle that lay directly under the skin. Use your fingers to press and knead along the centerline in the back of your calf.

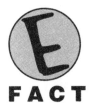

FACT

Shin splints, which is another name for inflammation of the tendons and muscles attached to the bone in the front of the lower leg, can cause pain. The tendons and muscles attached to this bone become inflamed often as a result of repetitive motion. Overexercising, running, walking up and down hills, or treadmill work may all produce this condition.

Using the pads of your fingers, press and circle down the front of your leg on each side of your shinbone. When you reach the ankle glide back to the top of your shin and repeat the circles.

Using both hands, press and glide deeply from your ankle up to your knee using your fingers. Press deeply over the entire front and sides of your lower leg, avoiding any pressure on the bone. Lastly, with both hands use your fingers to press deeply with horizontal lines from the ankle to the knee.

Switch legs and work the same routine on your other leg, starting with the gliding stroke over your calf, and kneading the back of your calf from your ankle to your knee.

Your Feet

You will massage the tops, sides, and bottoms of both your feet. Work one foot at a time in a sitting position with your foot crossed over your other leg. Start by pressing and kneading the sole of your foot with a wringing technique, using both hands. Use your thumbs to apply circular friction on the sole, as shown in **FIGURE 9-5**.

FIGURE 9-5

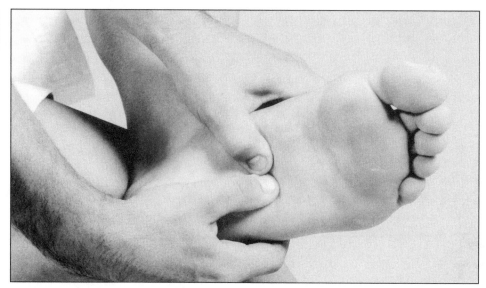

▲ Circular friction of the sole.

With one hand, press your fingers along the sole of your foot in imaginary lines from your heel to your toes. Press your fingers in, slowly moving up your foot. The arch of your foot may be sensitive so apply less pressure there.

Now, using both hands again, circle with your fingers around your ankle, pressing gently and firmly. Work around your entire ankle to the very back of your heel, which is a very sensitive region known as the Achilles heel; apply firm but gentle pressure there. Smooth the ankle area with circular gliding strokes that evolve into light feathering with just the tips of your fingers touching your ankle.

Next, grasp all your toes with one hand and gently squeeze them and release, applying slight pressure with the heel of your palm. As you stroke along each toe from the bottom to the tip of the nail, one toe at a time, pay attention to the pressure—it should be firm yet gentle. Work the top and bottom of each toe. Grasp all your toes again and gently squeeze. Lastly, stroke gently over the top and bottom of your foot in soft, feathering strokes. Move to your other foot and repeat, starting with pressing and kneading the sole.

Lower Back

This area includes the region below your rib cage to the back of your buttocks. Place both hands behind you, resting your hands between your ribs and your waist. This marks the kidney area. Move your hands down to your tailbone and begin to glide from the center of your body out to the side. Glide in and out as far as you comfortably can as you move up your lower back. Glide down and circle up, three times. Rest your hands at your waistline and knead in to either side of the spine.

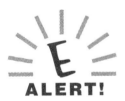

Remember; do not work directly on the spine. The vertebrae (the bones of the spine) house the spinal cord, from which all nerves emanate. Never press on this area. These small bones guard the operating system of the body. Massage providers do not adjust bones; chiropractors do.

Lift, pinch, and press along your waistline, moving down your back to your tailbone. Knead alongside your tailbone, moving out toward the upper curve of your hip. Knead back in and over the entire buttock area. Using an effleurage stroke, gently move up your lower back from your buttocks to the bottom of your rib cage.

Work from your rib cage to the side of your body, kneading as you go. Continue to knead from your spine out to the side to just below the waistline. Knead back and forth along this area at least three times. Use gentle gliding circles to complete your lower back.

Face, Head, and Neck

The tension of your daily life is often held in your head and neck and shows on your face. By massaging yourself in these areas you can release the built-up tension, relaxing your muscles, encouraging yourself to be restful. Massage in general, and working these areas in particular, helps you to slow down and be in the present moment. Healing touch is a gift that you are bringing to yourself.

To begin, place both your open hands gently on your face as you inhale and exhale. Let your hands rest here through three deep breaths. Circle your hands up and out over either side of your face, using your nose as the dividing line. Your entire palms and your fingers glide smoothly over your skin as you inhale on the up stroke and exhale on the circle out and down. Then use both your hands to glide up your neck from your chest, one hand following the other in long smooth strokes off the chin.

FIGURE 9-6

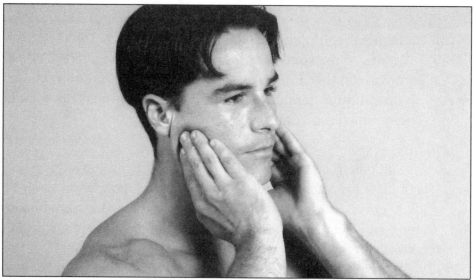

▲ Kneading stroke on the cheeks.

Now place both hands on the sides of your face, kneading with your fingers from your jaw to your cheeks. As you can see in **FIGURE 9-6,** your hands are pointing up toward your ears as your fingers knead your cheeks.

Continue to knead in small circles over your entire jaw and cheek area. You are releasing any tightness in your jaw as well as stimulating your gums.

Use the same circular kneading with your fingertips from the sides of your nose out to your ears and back again. Feel your sinuses begin to open as the muscles in this area loosen. Using gentle pressure, circle with your fingers from your eyes onto your forehead, making spiral patterns in lines running from your eyebrows out to the sides of your head,. Refer to **FIGURE 9-7** for the position of your fingers.

FIGURE 9-7

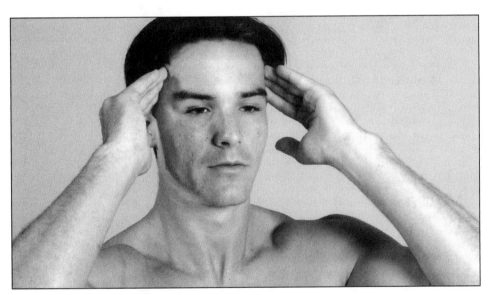

▲ Spiral strokes on the head.

Using all your fingers, move onto your scalp, circling with small tight strokes up from your forehead. Continue to use the small circle strokes as you work over your entire head, ending up at the bony ridge on either side of your neck at the base of your skull. Place your fingers into the notches on both sides of your neck, and make small circular movements.

Alternate your hands as you hold and squeeze gently on the back of your neck. Check your hand position by referring to **FIGURE 9-8**.

FIGURE 9-8

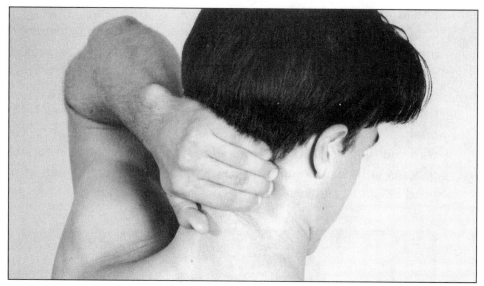

▲ Squeezing stroke on the back of your neck.

Feel the tightness releasing from your neck. Now place your fingertips back into the notches at the base of your skull, and press in and hold as you count to five. Slowly ease your fingers away as you glide down the back of your neck to your shoulders in sweeping strokes. Massage over your entire scalp and back of your neck again with small circular strokes, ending with the sweeping strokes off your shoulders.

Close with Chakras

The ancient Sanskrit word for wheel is chakra. Chakras are wheels, or circles, of energy that continuously spin in a gentle clockwise fashion, connecting to prominent areas of our bodies. The gentle massage you just gave yourself has affected your entire physical body, and at the same time has affected your chakras, balancing your emotions and your spiritual self. The loving kind touch you have experienced resounds throughout your entire being.

At this moment you are whole. Your intention to treat yourself with loving kindness has allowed you to release tension and experience a time of simple joy. You are a vital, loving person who has created a healing space within and without. Lie down comfortably if you are able, because this will allow you to totally experience this place you have created. Try to allow yourself to experience the full benefit of your massage.

Lying flat, close your eyes and breathe deeply. Rest your arms at your sides, palms up. Feel your breath cleansing and healing with every inspiration and expiration. Imagine your cleansing breath flowing through your body, pushing any toxins out through your palms and soles of your feet. Imagine now a strong healing heat flowing through your hands.

Place one hand flat on your pelvic region and the other hand just above it but below your belly button. Rest your hands gently, feeling the heat flow from your palms into your body. Empty your mind of busy thoughts and breathe. Think of a soft glowing red light flowing through your bottom hand. Feel its warmth. Through your top hand, imagine an orange light gently flowing into your body. Relax.

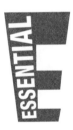

Breathing from the abdomen helps to release toxins from the body. Life-giving energy flows into the body through the nose, filling the lungs. The lungs send oxygen into the blood and take carbon dioxide out. As you exhale the lungs push the toxins out and the cycle continues.

Move your bottom hand up above your belly button and rest it palm down. Bring your other hand up into the center of your breastbone and place it gently there, palm down. Feel your body under your hands. Concentrate on the heat flowing between your hands and your body. Imagine a yellow light flowing out of the hand on your belly down into your stomach and beyond, spreading warm golden light. From the hand resting on your chest, imagine a brilliant green light radiating into your heart.

Take the hand from your stomach and rest it gently on your throat. Move the hand from your breastbone and rest it on your forehead. Now sense the energy flowing from your hands as the warmth increases. Imagine a sky-blue light flowing into your body from the hand resting on your throat. Imagine a deep indigo-blue light flowing between your eyes from the hand resting on your forehead. Feel these lights as they send soft and nurturing warmth. You are very relaxed yet vibrantly energized.

Now let both your hands rest for a moment on the top of your head. Imagine a deep violet light flowing from your hands down through your entire body. As the violet light moves into every part of you, rest your arms at your sides, palms up. Feel the peace that is flowing through your body. Enjoy it, embrace it, and remember it.

You have touched and awakened the healer within. Celebrate this part of yourself often. Remember to breathe and stretch. Remember to love yourself always. Enjoy the wonderfulness that is you with yourself and with others. When you are aware of your body, you become more aware of others. Massage yourself often. Massage others almost as much.

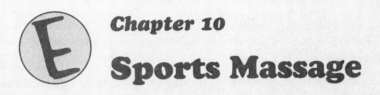

Chapter 10

Sports Massage

Athletes are trained muscle machines, although at times they seem to not pay attention to their training. Whether you are a professional athlete, a community or school sports player, or you work out on your own, you are an athlete. Sports massage helps to improve just about everything you do, so if you use your body you can benefit from it.

The Concept of Sports Massage

Whatever you do with your body, at whatever age you are, if you are physically active you will benefit from sports massage. Sports massage improves circulation and helps provide greater endurance. It also helps prevent injury by warming up the muscles, and helps repair injuries caused by repetitive use.

Sports massage can be administered during training for an event, before an event, and after an event. Sports massage protocol involves certain massage strokes, stretches, and injury-prevention exercises tailored to the sport and muscles used in the activity. After massage, athletes may be advised to use cold or hot compresses as well.

The competitive circumstances of athletes may be in the professional arena, or athletes may compete with themselves. By helping competitors stay injury free, sports massage gives them an edge over other participants. Sore muscles recover more quickly and become stronger and more supple when massaged. A massage before an event is a great way to warm up muscles, preparing the competitor for whatever activity she may be undertaking. Actually, sports massage could be renamed competitors' massage, because this describes who the massage is really for.

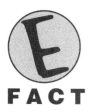

FACT

Sports massage has a multinational history. Although the idea of massage specifically for athletes originated in Greece, the techniques have a close connection with those used in Swedish massage. These techniques were further refined by sports trainers in Russia.

The Effects of Sports Massage

The massage geared toward the physically active has tremendous benefits. The obvious effect of sports massage is better performance, regardless of what it is you actually do with your body. Sports massage helps you reach your peak physically, by improving your circulation while keeping your muscles strong and flexible. Improved circulation reduces your chances of injury and allows for better overall movement.

Sports massage also warms up the muscles beyond whatever stretching you may do. It warms up muscles by stimulating the fleshy part of the muscle, called the belly. Working on the belly of the muscle promotes the distribution of oxygen throughout the entire muscle. Oxygen energizes the muscle, and waste products that interfere with muscle function are encouraged to leave the body through the blood and the lymph system.

Sports massage helps strengthen and tone your muscles and supports the nerves. The soothing effect massage has on the nerves helps promote a state of well-being, allowing you to perform at your best. As your nerves relax tension begins to release, giving you a chance to visualize yourself as a winner. Whether you are playing a sport for a national team, building a house, dancing on stage, or competing in a high school sport, your performance is important.

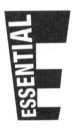

The condition known as ischemia, a deficiency of blood to a particular area, is a common side effect of physical exercise. This obstruction of blood flow causes pain or spasms in the muscle. If these spasms and soreness are not treated they can develop into chronic sites of pain. Left untreated, ischemia can even cause tissue death. Massage is an effective way to virtually eliminate this issue.

Sports massage works through the application of certain strokes by first relaxing the nerve receptors and then invigorating these same receptors through a different application of strokes. Depending upon the athlete's need, the massage can be both relaxing and stimulating, or only one of these. Sports massage is generally provided in a short, timed session that provides energy before an event or brings relaxation after an event. The improvement in soft tissue through this type of massage allows for better and longer performance, with less chance of injury and quicker recovery.

Techniques for Sports Massage

The various techniques employed in sports massage are derived from Swedish massage. The basic strokes are effleurage, petrissage, friction, stretching, and pressing, which you learned about in Chapter 5. These strokes are applied depending upon what the athlete needs from the massage. In this chapter you will learn which strokes to apply, for how long, and with what intensity, all in the context of sports massage.

Using Effleurage Strokes

Effleurage is the gliding stroke that flows over the body of the recipient. You use this stroke to smooth and warm up the body before you move in deeper. Remember to push toward the heart first and then pull back. You can see in **FIGURE 10-1** how your hands should rest, with your palms flat on the contours of the body and your wrists extended, not stiff or flexed.

FIGURE 10-1

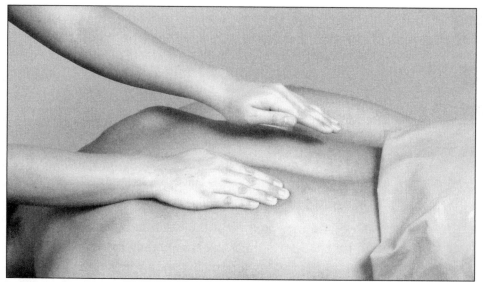

▲ Rest your hands with flat palms.

Effleurage may also be applied by making circles over the area you are working, which is a deeper movement. This circular stroke flushes out toxins and increases circulation in a smaller area. You may effleurage with either long, gliding strokes or tighter circles; either one helps prepare the receiver for all other massage work.

Using Petrissage Strokes

Following effleurage you might introduce the kneading application of petrissage. With this stroke you lift the tissue into your palm and knead or squeeze to release tension. This method works on the back and the thigh while smaller areas are more easily worked by using your fingers and thumbs.

Fulling is a petrissage technique that works well in sports massage. For this stroke you hold the flesh with both hands, push the underlying muscle up between your hands, and then stretch it back down away from the bone. Practice the fulling stroke on your thigh by placing both hands on either side of the thigh muscle and pushing the muscle up in the middle before stretching away on either side.

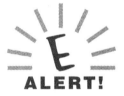

One of the biggest mistakes made by someone applying massage is to use his or her hands and fingers incorrectly. Do not bend at the joints. Your fingers should not bend in a sharp angle from your hands, and your hands should not bend in a sharp angle from your wrists. Hold your hands so that they flow into your arms, and keep your wrists flexible.

Skin rolling is another petrissage move that works well in sports massage. This stroke is applied by lifting the tissue up between your fingers and thumbs as you compress the tissue. Roll the skin between your fingers using both hands as you move along the area, lifting, pressing, and rolling. This technique may be painful at first so remember to ask your receiver if she is comfortable with your touch. This rolling helps loosen the connective tissue and release adhesions.

Petrissage also increases the blood flow and moves toxins up for release. It also helps release hormones that relieve pain, and it stimulates the nervous system as well. The release of tension with petrissage is deep, going in to the belly of the muscle. Muscle soreness and stiffness are reduced and sometimes eliminated with petrissage.

Using Friction Strokes

Friction applies heat to the underlying muscle while moving the top layer of skin over the deeper layers. Friction helps improve circulation within the tendons and ligaments, which are areas that generally do not receive much blood flow. The initial friction stroke is applied with your hands flat down on the body. Your hands move back and forth in two straight lines, passing each other in a continued movement along the surface being worked. The movement is steady with an increase in speed as you become accustomed to the body underneath.

Friction of the arm or leg is done by rolling or wringing the area between both hands in opposite directions. This is cross-fiber friction. You may friction the forearm or calf in this manner by bending the recipient at the elbow or knee and wrapping both your hands around the limb. **FIGURE 10-2** shows you how to position your hands and fingers to wring the muscles of the calf.

 FIGURE 10-2

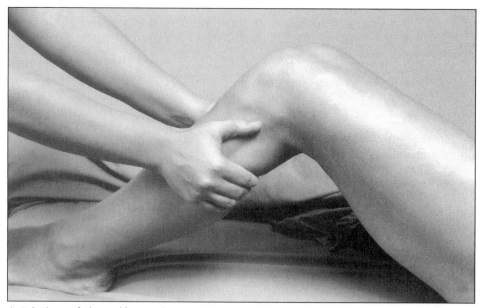

▲ Friction of the calf muscle.

Think of cross-fiber movements as small bites working their way across the muscle, as opposed to smooth, gliding movements up and down the muscle fibers or in-and-down pressing movements. Cross-fiber friction can be applied all over the body, including the extremities. Place your fingers on the area and firmly press in a back-and-forth motion.

Using Stretching

This is a combination of stretching the receiver and teaching the recipient how to stretch. Passive stretching by you helps to extend the muscle tissue without the owner of the muscle participating. You apply gentle pressure to allow the muscle to stretch a tiny bit farther than it could without your assistance. Effleurage provides some of this stretch because it loosens connective tissue. You may assist further with a simple guidance of the body part in the direction of the stretch.

In another form of assisted stretching, the receiver is an active participant. You allow the recipient to press or pull a muscle or group of muscles that you are holding. For example, hold the receiver's arm out straight in one hand and ask him or her to press down on your resisting hold; then reverse your hold and ask the receiver to press up into your hand. This type of stretch assists in developing strength and flexibility of the muscles.

Finally, encourage your athlete to follow a full regimen of stretching post-workout as well as warming up the muscles before an event or workout.

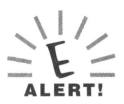

Warming up a muscle is very different from stretching. During warm-up the athlete should mimic in the warm-up moves the behavior of the activity he will be performing, such as walking on a treadmill before running. It is important to allow one's temperature and circulation to increase before moving into any activity, including stretching.

Stretching helps to relax and release sore muscles, allowing for quicker recovery. Stretching also helps by increasing muscle flexibility, mobility, and the flow of blood and oxygen as well.

Using Pressing

This method of massage is used to increase circulation and encourage the relaxation of the muscle. Pressing, or compression, helps to warm up the muscle, which helps an athlete prepare for activity. Position the palm of your hand on the muscle that needs attention, and apply pressure directly onto the belly of the muscle in a steady rhythmic motion. Place your other hand on top of the pressing hand to assist in the application of pressure. Remember not to bend at the wrist but to keep the hand loose.

If you encounter a muscle in spasm, apply even pressure without moving, keeping your hand on the spasm for a count of ten and then removing it. The compression and release will help reduce the spasm in the muscle. Under compression, a muscle produces a chemical that helps release the constriction.

Using Tapping

Tapping as part of a sports massage is performed with the sides of your hands or your fingers along the affected area. It is an invigorating technique that stimulates blood and oxygen flow, and is used to provide added energy, generally before an event. It provides a toning effect that helps to warm up the muscles.

When to Massage Athletes

The application of sports massage depends upon the needs of the individual athlete. Typically, it is most effective when used during training as well as during competition: before an event, after an event, and as maintenance long-term.

During Regular Training

During training you work to strengthen the athlete's muscles for endurance and injury prevention. Massage will enhance the athlete's performance and familiarize the receiver to sports massage technique.

The technique you use for the athlete in training is the same routine as any Swedish massage (see Chapter 18), with an emphasis on areas of the body that experience added stress due to the particular exercise, sport, or job the athlete participates in.

If the athlete is willing to continue massage even when not competing, she will reap its long-term benefits. Maintenance massage keeps the muscle healthy while dealing with any chronic soreness or pain.

Before an Event

Pre-event massage is used as an additional warm-up, providing an edge to the performance of the athlete. This massage is styled to provide stretch and movement by encouraging the flow of blood and oxygen to the muscles and loosening connective tissue. The athlete's body will respond more effectively due to the improved flexibility of the muscles, tendons, and ligaments. With improved flexibility, the joints become more mobile and the toxins are forced from the body.

Often overtraining can cause overly tight muscles and also mental tension. A ten-minute massage applied thirty minutes before an event will not only relieve tight, tense muscles, it will invigorate all the athlete's senses, providing a positive degree of readiness. Before an event do not use deep pressure and do not stay too long on one spot. The idea is to give added support physically, mentally, and emotionally through your massage.

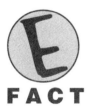

FACT

Our body works to stay in a state of balance, constantly working toward homeostasis. The trauma of damaged tissue sets a process in motion to let the body heal itself. Inflammation is the body's way of saying slow down and take a break. If the body heeds the message regeneration can occur.

After an Event

Massage after an event is a powerful implement in dealing with the aftereffects of a rigorous routine. The muscles in the participant's body have been pushed to the limit, causing the muscle tissue to swell. There may be soreness and inflammation depending upon the level of trauma the muscles have sustained. Immediately after an event most athletes experience some soreness due to the build up of waste resulting from the exertion. Such discomfort following exercise responds well to massage, and a thirty-minute massage after the event will help with these issues.

After an activity, sports massage helps to restore the muscles to their normal condition and helps the body to heal itself. The muscles that have experienced contraction and spasm begin to relax during massage as the toxins are pushed from the body. The high mental tension the performer maintained during the event is also released during massage as the body begins to relax.

Post-event becomes post-recovery as the body moves toward repair. If muscle soreness does not dissipate, continue working with the athlete on a weekly basis, addressing specific issues through a longer massage. As you work toward releasing soreness, your massage will teach the receiver's muscles to loosen and stretch naturally. Regular sports massage locates and removes chronic issues and helps the receiver become more aware of the needs and requirements of his or her body.

The more the participant understands the benefit of long-term massage, the better equipped the athlete will be to consistently perform well. Sports massage maintenance improves all aspects of the athlete's life by helping the athlete develop a pattern of injury-free living. Regular massage supports the heavy demands of the athlete's performance and enhances his or her ability to maintain strength and endurance.

Routines for Sports Massage

The routine for sports massage depends upon the athlete and what phase—training, pre-event, post-event—you are dealing with. Massage given during training is primarily a maintenance technique. Massage given before an event is energizing, while a massage given after the event is relaxing and healing. Generally sports massage is administered with little or no oil and the receiver stays clothed. Of course, any massage may be given this way.

Pre-Event Warm-Up for the Back of the Body

Given before a sports event, this massage provides the benefits of a warm-up and at the same time invigorates the mind and body, stimulating the systems to a state of complete readiness. To begin, have your receiver lie facedown, and then apply strong effleurage strokes in great sweeping movements over his or her back from the base of the spine up to the shoulders, and back around. Remember to move your body in a rocking motion as you apply these strokes, moving in toward the receiver on the up stroke and back from the receiver on the down stroke. Repeat this effleurage a number of times, using smooth, steady, firm pressure, and listen to your hands.

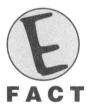

FACT

Sports massage activates the release of chemicals that reduce pain and promote relaxation. The production of stress hormones is reduced, allowing for better performance, and the production of "feel good" hormones is increased, supporting positive mental and emotional health.

Now apply compression on the back with a rhythmic pumping, moving up the back along the spine to the shoulders. Repeat this three or four times, pumping smoothly over the surface of the back. If the receiver indicates she has spasms in this area, press down on and hold the region (do not pump), and then release after the count of five. Finally, with your hands or just your fingers, use a tapping motion from the receiver's waist to the shoulders and down the back, providing stimulation to the muscles.

Next, knead over the buttocks as demonstrated in **FIGURE 10-3**, and then continue down the legs with a gliding stroke.

Apply an effleurage stroke up the legs from the ankles to the buttocks and back to the ankles. Using a friction stroke, start at the ankle and wring up the calf to the back of the knee and down to the ankle, repeating three or four times. At the top of the knee begin with a circling pressure stroke, and stroke up the leg to the hips and buttocks. Using petrissage, knead the hips and buttocks before turning the receiver over.

FIGURE 10-3

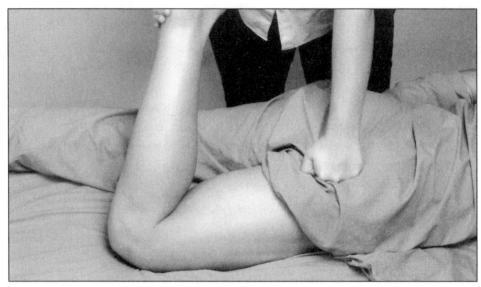

▲ Knead the buttocks.

Pre-Event Warm-Up for the Front of the Body

With the recipient lying on his or her back, start the front massage of the arms and legs. Begin on the right arm and effleurage from the wrist to the shoulder and back again, three times. Apply a rolling stroke along the arm, lifting it when necessary to reach all parts of the arm. Bend the arm at the elbow and wring it from the wrist to the elbow and back again. With both your hands, stretch the right hand on both sides. Now, starting with the recipient's arm at his or her side, parallel to the body, use both your hands to carefully stretch the arm out to the side, and up alongside the recipient's ear, then back through to the recipient's side. Repeat on the left arm.

Move to the left leg and effleurage in long sweeping strokes up from the ankle to the hip and down, three to five times. Then wring up from the ankle to the knee, and repeat three times. Next lift and roll the thigh muscles up to the hips using a kneading stroke, and repeat three times.

Move back to the recipient's feet and, using both hands, stretch the left foot on the top and the bottom. After the stretch, rest both hands on the top of the left foot with your thumbs reaching across the sole. Wring up and down the foot as demonstrated in **FIGURE 10-4**.

FIGURE 10-4

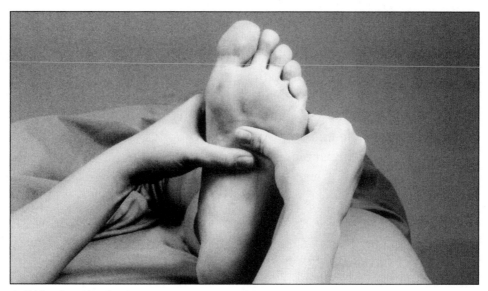

▲ Wringing the foot.

Repeat your massage on the right leg, starting with effleurage from the ankle to the hip, and ending with wringing the right foot. Complete the leg massage by tapping each leg from the ankle to the hips.

Post-Event Massage

It is best to provide massage as soon as possible following an event, because waste products may have built up during an activity, and these can cause sore, painful, and sensitive muscles. Post-event massage helps to prevent stiffness and fatigue, and helps the athlete to relax.

Begin with the receiver lying on his or her stomach, and effleurage the entire back from the waist to the shoulders and back to the waist. Then gently glide up the recipient's arm, from the hand to the neck and back to the hand. Repeat three times on each arm before moving to the legs. Now glide up the thigh from the back of the knee, over the buttocks and down through the hips back to the knee. Finally, effleurage from the ankle to the back of the knee and down to the ankle. Repeat three times, with each glide becoming deeper, then move on to the other leg.

As your hands glide over the body, can you feel what areas are tense? More than likely the legs hold most of the tension, followed by the back or neck. The next part of the massage is designed to relieve this tension in the legs. Begin with fulling of the hamstrings by placing both your hands on either side of the left thigh, just above the back of the knee. Press in to push up the muscle, and then stretch out the skin to the sides. Perform this fulling technique up the back of the leg to the top of the thigh, and repeat moving down to your starting position, just above the back of the knee.

Carefully knead along the entire back of the thigh from the knee to the buttock and back again. Stroke gently over the back of the knee and continue kneading the entire calf muscle, if this move feels fine to the recipient. Then, using friction, pinch and roll the calf from the ankle to the knee, stopping just below the soft area behind the knee. Use this pinch-and-roll friction down the calf and back up to the knee, repeating this stroke twice more.

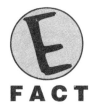

FACT

After an event, massage should not cause more pain to muscles that are already sore. If after the initial touch the receiver complains of pain, move on from that area. Application of pressure too soon after a sporting event will only cause more stress, and will not allow the muscle to heal.

Wring up the left leg from the ankle to the knee, stroke over the knee, and knead up to the top of the thigh. Standing to the left side of the person makes this move easy. Now place your hands on the left buttock, one hand on top of the other, with the heel of your palm pressing into the buttock. Press release, press release, and press and hold, feeling the buttock relax. Next, stand at the recipient's feet, hold the left leg by the calf, and bend the leg into the buttock as far as the leg will easily go. Do not force the stretch. Slowly release the leg and repeat the entire procedure on the right leg, starting with the fulling of the right thigh.

This basic post-event routine can be used on any area of the body that is feeling stress from the activity. Make sure the recipient drinks plenty of water to flush out the toxins and metabolic waste your massage work released from the muscles and other organs. In addition to releasing built-up toxins, the post-event massage jump-starts the blood and lymph flow. Remind your receiver to breathe and stretch after the massage is over.

Understanding Sports Injury

Dedicated athletes often work in pain, and it becomes part of their lives. Athletes will not generally stop training and competing, but instead make the conscious choice to work through the pain. Your job is to educate the recipient on the tissue damage such behavior generates (see Chapters 8 and 16). Explain how the damage affects the healing time and the concept of chronic pain. Once you have presented these ideas, you have made your position clear, and the choice to continue remains with the recipient. Allow the performer to make an educated decision from your information, as you remain clear that your intention is to provide healing as needed.

Overloading

Athletes often try to improve their performance by training with a technique known as overloading. The idea is that the more you do the more you challenge your cardiovascular system and muscles, and the more you improve your performance. The other part of this idea is that the body must rest and recover in order for you to continue reaching for added challenge. Sometimes athletes do too much too fast and do not allow their bodies sufficient time to recover between challenges. Then they end up with overuse injuries.

The damage caused by overuse may result in a variety of injuries to the soft tissue of the body. Massage is an important tool in the repair of this damage. Muscle soreness is the most frequent complaint and is associated with a small degree of pain and perhaps spasms. Effleurage, compression, and petrissage are good techniques for this type of injury.

Strains and Sprains

Strains and sprains are injuries often caused by quick movements or by muscle soreness that is ignored. When such an injury occurs in a muscle, it is called a strain; when it occurs in a ligament, it is called a sprain. The tearing of tissue and the resulting scarring can be painful. Whichever injury is sustained, initially the swelling and pain must subside somewhat before massage can be used. Friction massage is helpful in working with the scars that form under the skin as the tissue repairs itself.

Sports massage can help anyone who is active. If you use your body for more than sitting you can benefit from all aspects of this type of massage. Children can benefit from shorter sessions, because often they cannot remain still for the full sessions. Anyone you know who needs some rest and restoration can benefit from sports massage. Ⓔ

... of Chair Massage

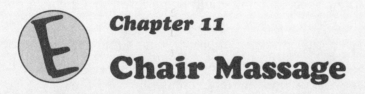

Chapter 11

Chair Massage

Chair massage has allowed the field of touch to enter into the office, the airport, sports events, concerts, malls, and the offices of medical professionals. You will find chair massage therapists volunteering their services during medical disasters and emergencies. The relaxation and pain relief experienced from a ten- to twenty-minute seated massage promotes a sense of well-being and productivity that has surpassed all expectations.

Evolution of Chair Massage

Early massage therapists in the United States were trained in many modalities, including shiatsu, anma, and trigger-point therapy, bodywork techniques practiced by Eastern cultures since ancient times. These therapies, although not technically massage, were required subjects for practitioners of massage, and all could by performed, at least in part, with the recipient in a seated position. Massage therapists developed new techniques based on this seated approach, and some early therapists brought these techniques into the workplace, offering a professional, seated massage to employees in large companies.

Massage schools began to recognize the variety of uses that seated massage could provide and developed curricula to service that need. In the late 1970s a massage professional demonstrated her seated technique to attendees at a national massage conference, sparking interest in this method. As a result, training programs in massage began to reflect the variety of populations served by massage, including seated massage, and eventually established a protocol for seated massage, which allows the service to be offered to everyone, regardless of physical restrictions.

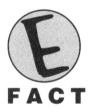

FACT

Seated massage has origins that can be traced to ancient China. More than 3,000 years ago, the Chinese discovered points that trigger healing responses when touched. This discovery spread throughout the Eastern world, influencing healing work in Japan and India as well. Many of these traditional styles included a form of seated massage as part of the treatment.

Educators, parents, and massage therapists, realizing the value of seated massage, began to look for and develop programs offering this technique. Populations of less-able children and adults began to receive this style of massage. And employees in large corporations were encouraged to take advantage of corporate-sponsored chair massages. Progress had caught up with the practice of easing our tired backs by rubbing them on a chair.

Chair Massage Today

A massage therapist named David Palmer worked to promote chair massage during the early 1980s. At first Palmer's group had a minimal amount of success promoting his chair-massage service to the business world. However, in 1984 Palmer acquired Apple Computer as a client, and the chair-massage practitioners found their niche. Through Palmer's innovative work, chair massage is no longer a mystery. Today, this accessible method of massage is relaxing hundreds of people daily, not only in the workplace but also in countless other arenas.

Unlike traditional massage, which is generally private, chair massage is very visible, so people can observe what takes place and know what to expect if they decide to try it. It has taken the mystery and fear out of bodywork, plus it is easy to receive and it is inexpensive. For many folks, chair massage is their introduction into the healing world of skilled, compassionate touch.

In the Office or on the Road

Chair massage offers a time-saving and inexpensive approach to stress relief. This approach to massage offers a welcome break, without caffeine or nicotine! Recipients of chair massage do not have to worry about being undressed, either. Although skilled, compassionate touch is wonderful, many people feel uncomfortable undressed or partially undressed, even draped with a cover. Chair massage offers a healthy alternative and an acceptable introduction into the remarkable world of massage.

Corporate Massage

The introduction of chair massage into the world of fast pace, fast money, and fast demands has provided a remarkable doorway for change within the corporate setting. The work ethic of most Americans is work until you drop, providing your company with the best output you can produce. The integrity of most workers is impeccable and deserves to be rewarded, as most owners of companies realize.

Chair massage provides a healthy break from the stress of the workplace. Fortunately, many companies realize the benefits of massage to their employees and the resulting increase in overall production, so they have introduced on-site chair massage. The brief time an employee spends receiving the massage reaps incredible rewards for both the employee and the company.

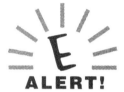

ALERT!

Any part of the body that repeats the same motion over a period of time may develop a strain in the muscles. This painful condition limits mobility and restricts the use of the injured area until the muscle repairs. Muscles that stay in one position for an extended period of time can also develop strain and tension. Chair massage helps to prevent these injuries.

Imagine a busy office, with phones ringing, fax machines whirring, computer screens glaring, and a five o'clock deadline. Everyone is anxious and unhappy; worry lines are present on many foreheads. Now is the time for you to introduce the chair massage routine you have been studying. You enlist the help of your closest associate and begin by turning her chair so the back faces her desk. You pull out a small travel pillow from your bottom drawer and place it on the top of the chair back.

Your partner in adventure straddles the chair, resting her head on the pillow, her arms on her knees. You place your hands on her shoulders, palms down, getting ready to begin. By now everyone starts to notice as you work on your fellow employee. She visibly relaxes as you follow a simple routine. The next recipient is already waiting as you finish with a few stimulating moves.

The healthy, upbeat changes this small routine makes in the overall attitude of your fellow workers will amaze you. On-site corporate massage provides a restful yet invigorating release of tension, creating an atmosphere of camaraderie that promotes resourcefulness and productivity. Don't forget to have someone work on you!

Travel Massage

Massage on the road is made easy with a seated routine. You can turn anything that can be sat on into a tool for massage. Folks who travel either for business or pleasure can give each other seated massage using a stool, a portable camping chair, or a blanket on the ground. Anyone can massage your shoulders and neck, releasing tension and stored energy while freeing stiff muscles and helping rid your body of toxins that may cause pain.

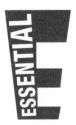

Chair massage has no added expense, because you do not have to buy oils or use linens to drape. You can buy a chair if you wish but it is not necessary. Remember to stretch after you give the massage to release any tension you may have created doing the work.

Other Environments

The opportunities available to provide chair massage are endless. Conventions and meeting centers are great places to offer chair massage. Charity events love to offer it as a great fundraising gift. Hospitals use chair massage for their staff, providing a calm and quiet space for the healers to be healed. No matter the profession, just about everyone is willing to try a chair massage. Truck drivers and construction workers receive tremendous benefits, as do the operators of buses and trains. Wait staff and dishwashers, cooks and bartenders, anyone who uses his or her body will love chair massage.

Advantages of Chair Massage

Massage of any type is fantastic, but there are many people who do not want to take off their clothes, never mind the part about lying on a table with their faces down, waiting for someone they don't know to rub them with oil. Even if the person giving the massage is a dear friend, some folks just don't like to get undressed. Chair massage recipients are fully clothed and sit in a chair while the giver targets areas of tension without using oil. The giver of the massage either brings a chair made for chair massage or improvises with whatever chair is available, so no one has to lie down on a table. Because the recipient is fully clothed and in a less vulnerable position than in traditional massage, this technique may even help eliminate someone's fear and worry of being touched.

Others can't seem to justify taking an hour solely for themselves. Chair massage, although highly effective, is brief, perhaps fifteen to twenty minutes, and can be done on a coffee break. Chair massage is usually conducted out in the open, which reinforces the feeling of safety in those who are somewhat timid. Massage given in the workplace lowers stress and, as a result, the number of stress-related illnesses. It also promotes a sense of well-being, and ultimately helps raise productivity.

Techniques for Chair Massage

The strokes used in chair massage are a combination of Eastern acupressure and Swedish massage techniques. You will use a combination of acupressure, compression, friction, stretching, petrissage, effleurage, tapping, and feather strokes, all applied through the clothes without oil. Your goal is to release the tension that can sit in the back, shoulders, neck, hands, and arms, releasing muscle stress and congestion. Overall you will be providing relaxation.

Using Acupressure and Compression

Acupressure is the application of pressure to an affected area for the purpose of releasing congested fluid buildup from the tissues and stretching the muscle. The pressure is applied and held on a spot by your finger, thumb, or both, or sometimes all your fingers. Holding on a point helps to break up muscle spasms. This stroke works in conjunction with friction and kneading petrissage.

Compression can also be applied with the heels of your hands in a steady, even, press-and-hold technique. Mold your hand to the part of the body being massaged, and press down firmly with the heel of your palm. Hold for a moment, release, and press again, moving in small increments over the area being worked.

Using Friction

Friction is the movement of skin over muscle, and can be applied in a variety of styles. One way is to place both your hands on the area, palms down, and move back and forth in a sliding movement over the region. This quickly warms up the muscles underneath. Use this movement along either side of the spine, on the broad area of the back, along the shoulders, or up the arms.

Another way to apply friction is more of an isolating move. Rather than gliding across the skin, press your fingers into the muscles, hold, and push the skin over the muscles as you move your fingers. By pressing you are able to reach in deeper. As you become more familiar with this movement, you can actually feel the muscle underneath. This type of friction works well with acupressure, because it allows you to focus on specific pressure points.

Using Stretching

There are three ways to use stretching in chair massage. One way is an active assisted stretch, which means you help your partner stretch a tiny bit more. For example, gently pull the receiver's arm as she stretches to open up the shoulder a little more. Another is an active resisted stretch, which means your partner resists the stretch as you gently pull. And the last one is the passive stretch, which means you do all the stretching while the person being worked on lets it happen. Be careful; do not push or pull aggressively. The passive stretch should be a smooth, gentle stretch that helps the muscle loosen. Pull gently, stop, and check with the receiver to see if the stretch is within her comfort range.

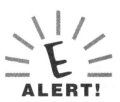

ALERT!

Be careful when you apply any stretching technique—move only as far as the joint will allow. The range of motion for any joint is how far it will stretch in any direction without causing discomfort. Do not move past that limit or you will injure your partner.

Using Petrissage

Petrissage is the kneading, rolling, twisting, squeezing, lifting, and pinching technique that gets in and breaks up the congestion. Petrissage can be applied in a number of ways. One style is deep kneading with the hands, which begins by lifting the flesh up into the palms and squeezing, using your fingers to push the skin. Lift, roll, and squeeze, grasping the flesh as you move along the area as one hand pushes the flesh in, and the other hand does the squeezing.

Another common petrissage technique is pinching with your thumb and fingers. Pick up the skin between your thumb and fingers, and roll along as your thumb pushes more flesh in to your fingers that are pinching in a constant rock-and-roll motion. Although it is important to move your body as you apply any massage stroke, kneading in particular feels better when combined with your body movement.

Using Effleurage and Feather Touch

Effleurage is used in chair massage to begin and end the session, as well as to assess the underlying tension. How firmly you glide depends on the "eyes" in your hands to feel and find where to glide deeper and where to stroke lightly. To glide more deeply, mold your hands to the body as you press along the surface in a smooth, rhythmic motion. To glide with a soft, feather touch gently brush your fingertips or palms along the region to calm the nerves. Effleurage may be used over most parts of the body and is especially great with chair massage because your hands can glide easily over clothing.

Using Tapotement

Tapotement in the form of tapping is useful in chair massage for the neck, head, and shoulders. Use your fingers to tap with either light or heavy pressure in these areas—either one feels good. Hacking (karate chops) works wonders on a tight back. Remember to keep your wrists loose and your hands limp, letting the sides of your hands and fingers do the work. You can also apply tapping with a loose fist, easily tapping over a broad surface. Cupping with your hands and tapping over the entire back provides added stimulation. Tapping is best applied by establishing a rhythm and moving over the area in time with the steady beat you have chosen.

A Chair Massage Routine

Remember, you do not have to buy a chair to give someone a chair massage. Simply turn a straight-back chair around and use a pillow on the back for the receiver to rest his or her head. You could also use a piano stool in front of a table. Place your partner on the stool with his or her head and arms resting on a pillow on the table. Piano or drummer stools are great because you can adjust the height to fit the person.

Begin the massage by leaning in toward the upper back and pressing your hands down on the shoulders as shown in **FIGURE 11-1**.

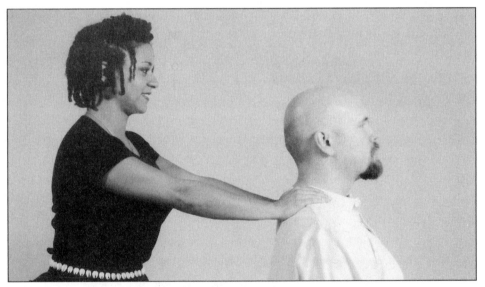

▲ Begin by greeting the recipient.

Press down with your palms and glide along the shoulder line out to the tops of the arms. Repeat this gliding stroke pressing down and away, relaxing the neck and shoulders. Lift and squeeze the flesh from the neck across the shoulders in a kneading stroke. As you can see in **FIGURE 11-2,** both hands are kneading together.

FIGURE 11-2

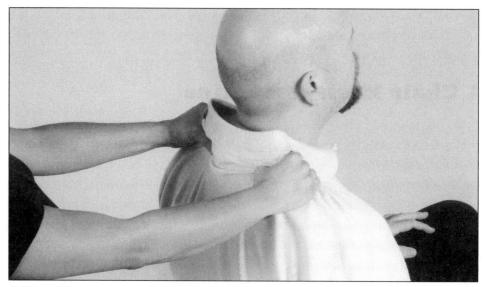

▲ Kneading the upper shoulders.

Return to the top of the neck, placing the first two fingers of each hand into the notch on either side of the spine at the base of the skull. Press down alongside the spine, using steady acupressure strokes, all the way to the lower back, as you see in **FIGURE 11-3**. Do not press on the spine.

FIGURE 11-3

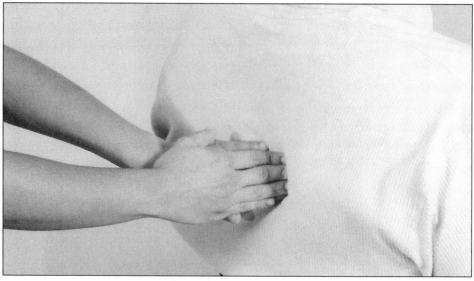

▲ Acupressure stroke along the side of the spine.

Return to the shoulders again and place one palm flat on the shoulder blade while you press down along the opposite side of the spine with two fingers. Repeat this technique on the other side and remember to move your body.

Lean in toward the receiver as you hold one shoulder with your forearm while you circle with friction over the other side of the back from the recipient's shoulders to the hips. Holding the opposite shoulder allows you to stabilize muscle and stretch the skin on the other side. Switch to the other side and repeat.

The Arms

Stand in front of the chair as you hold the recipient's arm with both hands. Rest the arm on your forearm as you glide over the entire arm with your other hand, turning it so you can touch all parts. Using both your hands, squeeze up and down the arm, stimulating the muscles. Next, use one hand to knead along the muscles of the upper arm, again supporting the arm with your other hand. You can see in **FIGURE 11-4** how one hand does the work while the other supports the arm.

FIGURE 11-4

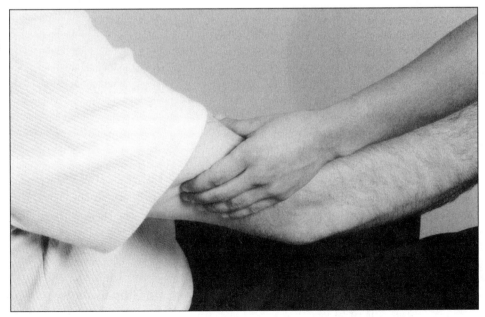

▲ Kneading the upper arm.

Now hold the arm under the elbow and under the wrist, and stretch. Remember to stop before you feel resistance. Then gently shake the arm, and feel the muscles relax. While you are holding the receiver's hand, press down the length of each finger and circle around the wrist. Remember not to pull the fingers, but rather support the wrist and slowly walk with your thumb down every finger. Refer to **FIGURE 11-5** to check your position when working on the hand.

Return the arm gently to your partner's side and repeat these strokes on the other arm.

FIGURE 11-5

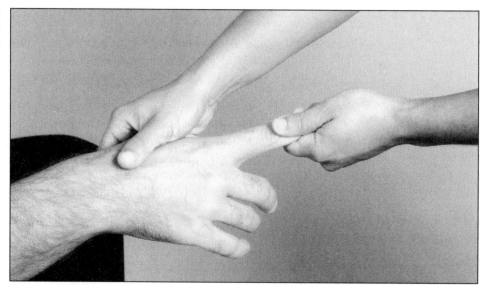

▲ Thumb walk down the finger.

Hips and Lower Back

When working on the lower back and hips you may find that kneeling or squatting works best for you. Lightly glide both hands down the recipient's back from the neck to the hips, two or three times. Then press along the side of the spine with your thumbs or fingers, starting below the rib cage and working right to the hip bones. Now move out from the center of the back and press along the buttocks out to the sides of the hips. Continue this pressing move, returning to the center and circling out until you have covered the entire lower back and hips.

Next use your palms and press into the lower back and all along the buttocks and hips. The heels of the palms will do most of the work with your fingers gliding along. Move each hand away from the center, pressing out.

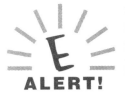

ALERT!

Remember to keep an ongoing check with your receiver. Whenever you move to a new section of the body ask how the pressure is and how the recipient is feeling overall. When trying something new, go slowly, keeping within the comfort range of the receiver.

For this next movement, work one side of the body and then the other. Again you will need to kneel or squat as you press with your thumbs or fingers along the side of the thigh from the hip to the knee. Press up and down along the thigh from the knee to the hip, working to the center of the thigh. Repeat these acupressure strokes back out to the side of the leg, then feather off. Move to the other leg and follow the same steps.

The Neck and Head

Standing behind the receiver, place both hands on either side of the receiver's neck and glide down and off the shoulders, using steady smooth pressure. Follow this by pressing two fingers in at the base of the skull and pressing to the bottom of the neck. Return your fingers to the top of the neck and press down again until you have covered the entire neck. Ask your receiver if the pressure is fine or if you need to ease up a bit.

Next, knead the neck by lifting and squeezing the neck muscles with one hand, pushing the flesh into your palm with your thumbs as you squeeze with your fingers, as shown in **FIGURE 11-6**.

Move down to knead the neck muscles that flow into the back. These hold a tremendous amount of tension. Finally, gently stretch the neck by holding one side at the top of the shoulder and gently guiding the stretch by a slight press to the head, as you can see in **FIGURE 11-7**. Stretch the neck to the left side and back to the center, and then over to the right side and back to the center again.

FIGURE 11-6

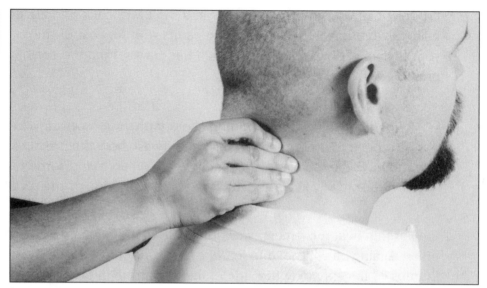

▲ Kneading the neck.

FIGURE 11-7

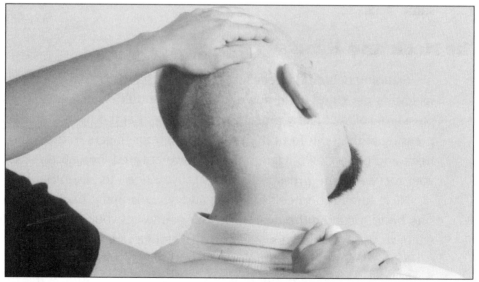

▲ Neck stretch.

Massage the scalp and hair with both hands using circular friction. The tips of your fingers act as though you are shampooing the head of your receiver. The movement is firm without gliding as your fingers lift from each section and move to the next. Then place your hands firmly on the head and gently knead by pressing in and moving the entire palm as you move gently over the entire scalp. Kneading is a great stroke to relieve slight pressure in the head. **FIGURE 11-8** shows you exactly how to hold your hands.

FIGURE 11-8

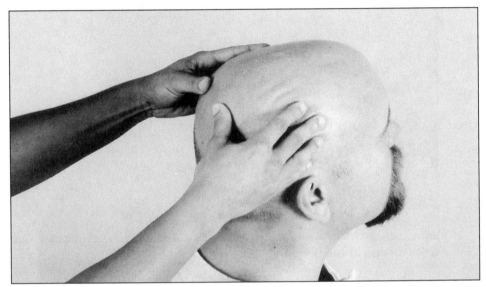

▲ Kneading the head.

The Finish

Tapping over the entire area you just massaged helps to announce the finish as well as invigorates the receiver. Begin with finger tapping from the receiver's head down to the buttocks and over the arms. Then, with your fists slightly closed, beat a gentle percussion stroke over the receiver's back and shoulders as shown in **FIGURE 11-9**.

Next, cup and slap each shoulder and arm with a steady beat, and follow this stroke onto the thighs. Glide your palms smoothly down both sides of the back; then press both your palms firmly on the shoulders, signaling the end.

Chair massage is fun. You can provide this type of a massage anywhere at just about any time. The routine can be changed, added to, or taken away from, depending upon what the needs are at the time. You can use this type of a massage to interest any of your friends and family who don't feel comfortable getting undressed. This is a great introduction into the relaxing world of massage.

FIGURE 11-9

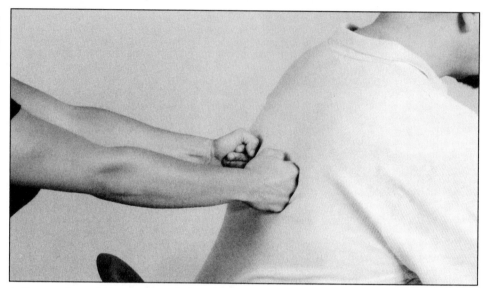

▲ Percussion of the back and shoulders.

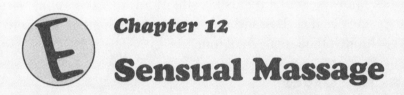

Chapter 12
Sensual Massage

Humans are sentient beings who feel and perceive through all of the senses. To be in touch with your body means that you are aware of the body that you live in—that you know the sensual feeling of being at home with yourself. To know your body is to be in harmony, aware of the connection between your body, mind, and soul. As you honor yourself so you honor others through the sharing of touch, the sensual sense.

Massage and Intimacy

Intimacy is the detailed knowledge you share with someone that is the result of a long or close association, such as the relationship you have with yourself, your family, or your romantic partner. Any loving, compassionate touch is intimate. To touch with tenderness communicates an intimate knowledge that needs no other form of expression. Massage speaks volumes as the giver and the receiver participate in an exchange of energy through the language of touch.

The Role of the Giver

As the giver, you are involved in one of the most delightful experiences of life, the joy of giving pleasurable touch. Through massage you give your partner a time of relaxation, a time to release all stress and to feel free, light, and alive. This is a time of listening through your hands as the silent language from your massage partner guides your hands to areas of tension and pain. You create a warm, safe atmosphere that allows your receiver to let go, allowing you to create a relaxing rhythm of pleasurable sensation.

The Role of the Receiver

To receive is an essential component of intimacy. Many people find it hard to give up control, to let someone else be in charge, and therefore find it easier to give than to receive. Letting go is a journey along the road of trust; to receive in massage is to accept quietly. The delicious sensations that radiate through your body when you are the receiver are to be enjoyed without reservation. Relish the silent space, think of nothing, and float freely. Be still, be at peace, and breathe.

The Benefits of Sensual Relaxation

Taking a walk together, holding hands, meditating, or giving each other a massage are all forms of relaxation that enhance the senses. Relaxing with a loved one in the privacy of your bedroom, a fancy suite, or a bed-and-breakfast by the sea feeds the senses. The intimacy of time spent together alone enhances your relationship. Quiet time together strengthens the bonds of loving trust, developing a shared experience that is unique to the connection between you and your partner.

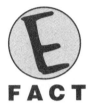

FACT

Relaxing calms the autonomic nervous system, the part of the nervous system that deals with blood pressure, breathing, and even your heartbeat. As you relax, your breathing slows, your blood pressure stabilizes, and your heart beats at a quieter pace.

To relax is to relieve the pressures of daily living and let go of your worries. True relaxation allows you to consciously release stress and tension, and sharing this release strengthens your intimate relationship. Spending time in sensual relaxation with your intimate partner provides an excellent way to reconnect. Together you can enjoy the voyage of exploration as you try the various techniques that deal with relaxation.

Muscle Relaxation

Progressive muscle relaxation and deep breathing help you and your partner relax quickly and deeply. The process of progressive muscle relaxation is easy. Lie on the floor and cover yourselves with a light blanket to ensure you stay warm. Close your eyes and lie with your hands open, palms facing up. Begin by tensing your toes and feet; tense and hold the muscles and release. Move up to your calf muscles; tense, hold, and release. Move up to your thighs and tense the muscles; hold and release. Continue to follow the tense-hold-release pattern as you work every muscle group all the way up your body. Finish with your face muscles; tense, hold, release; and then relax your whole body.

During this exercise breathe freely and deeply; do not hold your breath. When you have completed relaxing your muscles, allow yourself to savor the tranquil moment in peace and harmony with yourself and your partner. Practicing this technique together will help you and your romantic partner reach a state of deep relaxation faster each time you practice. Progressive muscle relaxation has a cumulative effect, meaning the more you do it, the better the effects.

Eating as Relaxation

Eating together in a calm, unhurried atmosphere is sensual. Dining together you experience a cornucopia of sights, smells, tastes, and textures that surprise and please the palate. Food provides energy but also makes you feel good. A beautifully arranged plate of healthy food provides a visual and olfactory experience long before you actually eat the food. Food is to be enjoyed, especially in company with each other.

A yogurt sundae invented by massage therapist and yoga teacher Tina Walsh is an explosion of sensual stimulation. Her recipe is simple. Layer the following ingredients in a large bowl:

- One cup natural granola
- Two cups vanilla yogurt
- One pint of cut strawberries
- One handful of walnuts
- A healthy sprinkle of shredded coconut

Use two spoons and enjoy together! You can create your own food specialties by improvising with foods you both enjoy.

Listen to Your Partner

In any relationship listening is key. To listen is to show honor and respect, to value the other. Everyone knows someone who shows support through the ability to listen well without interruption. Think of how you feel when you have someone's undivided attention. The feeling you experience is generally one of empowerment. In sensual massage it is important to listen to your partner before, during, and after the massage. Hear what your partner is saying through his or her words and sounds, and through your hands—pay attention and you will hear what your massage partner needs.

Listening with Your Ears

Before you actually massage each other, talk. Share how you feel physically and emotionally, and make sure that each of you wishes to be involved with touching at this time. Listen if your partner expresses complaints about physical aches and pains or emotional, mental, or spiritual worries. Your touch can help healing in any of these problem areas.

Always respect one another's wishes. If your partner does not feel like being touched today, do not force the issue. Remember times when you did not want to be touched and honor the desires of your partner. Compassionate touch is too important to force or insist; instead give a rain check.

Listening with Your Hands

Your hands provide another way of listening—they will allow you to hear more than the spoken word. Enlist your partner in an exercise of hand listening. Begin by sitting opposite each other, feet firmly planted on the floor, knees touching. Rest your hands on your thighs, and begin deep rhythmic breathing.

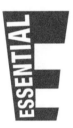

Proper breathing comes from deep within your belly. Inhale slowly, bringing your breath as far into your body as you can, feeling your chest expand. Hold your breath in for a moment, tightening your abdomen. Slowly release your breath, feeling your lungs empty and your stomach naturally pull in.

Listen to your own body first; close your eyes and place your hands on your shoulders and feel the muscles underneath your fingers. Are your shoulders tight, or do they feel relaxed? Take turns feeling each other's shoulders. How do they feel? Take your time getting a clear feeling of the body resting under your hands, whether it is yours or your partner's. Take turns feeling each other's arms. Are the upper arms taut and the lower arms loose, or vice versa? Listen to each other, feeling places of stress and tension. This exercise helps you to become more aware of your body and your partner's.

Setting the Stage for Sensual Massage

You have both decided you would like to give and receive a massage, and you have the time right now. The next step is to create a loving space that is inviting and sensual. Decide whether you want to set up a comfy spot on the floor, or use your bed or a table. Whatever you decide to use make sure the room is warm, with no drafts to create a chill. A light fleece blanket or flannel sheet adds the right amount of warmth without a heavy feeling. The lighting should be comfortable, not glaring.

Oil and Oil-Scented Candles

Today's marketplace has entire areas dedicated to the art of sensuality. There are many oils and oil-scented candles that you and your massage partner may want to experiment with. A common scent is Ylang Ylang oil from flowers of the Mediterranean that induces a feeling of well-being. Patchouli is an old favorite made from leaves of plants grown in Asia, India, and the West Indies. The scent of patchouli in oil or candles produces a calming and uplifting energy. Vetiver is a rich and woody scent from roots of plants from India and Haiti. This scent provides a strong calming sensation.

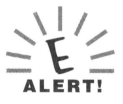

ALERT!

There are many scented candles that provide an exotic fragrance to a room. But not every scent appeals to everyone, so choose candles with your partner, picking scents that you both like. Whatever candles or oils you choose, discontinue use if either of you feels nausea or dizziness.

Quiet

Quiet is essential; shut off all phones, televisions, and radios. Ideally all children, pets, and other adults are either sleeping or not around. If you have some relaxing, soothing, instrumental music fine; otherwise, no music is good, too. To give and receive massage is fun; it is joyful if the setting is correct. Of course you can massage in the living room with everyone watching television, but that is a group event, not a sensual experience. Be clear on what you each expect so there are no interruptions.

Techniques for Sensual Massage

The massage techniques you have learned so far can all be used in a sensual massage. Discuss what you have time for or what you both feel like doing and proceed from there. You can spend an hour or twenty minutes—the time spent is not as important as the quality of your touch. Before you start, position the body of your receiver and drape him or her with a light cover.

While you are giving, keep your thoughts focused on the needs and desires of your partner; be attuned to what he enjoys and what is painful. Modulate your voice so it flows with the calmness of your touch, creating a warm, inviting experience. Establish a rhythm that is comfortable, allowing you to flow and glide with your movements, creating a symphony on your receiver's body. Use enough oil so that you can move easily over your partner's muscles with smooth strokes. Be sure to warm the oil between your hands, or you can place the container of oil in hot water first to warm it and keep it warm during use.

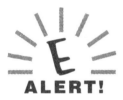

If a movement is painful do not repeat it. Always keep checking in, assuring your massage partner that you are attentive to his or her needs. If a pain persists even when not touched, don't attempt to massage at all; stop and consult a medical professional.

The main strokes that you use in any massage are effleurage (gliding), petrissage (kneading and compression), tapotement (tapping and percussion), and friction. You can apply these strokes at various times during sensual massage, depending upon what is needed. Your rhythm should be comfortable and smooth, and your strokes will flow over the body beneath you.

Using Effleurage and Petrissage

Effleurage is the circular stroke that glides over the surface, stimulating the flow of blood and oxygen while promoting the flow of lymph throughout the body. Petrissage is the kneading stroke that moves deeper into the muscle to stretch it and also increase blood flow. Both of these strokes are the mainstay of your massage, allowing light or deep penetration depending upon what is needed in the area you are working on. Use enough oil to allow freedom of movement and pay attention to areas that may need more oil because they are dry or have more hair.

When using effleurage, mold your hands to the shape of the receiver's body as you glide over the surface, and then press down with deeper and firmer strokes. Your movements follow the shape of the body you are working on, exploring the hills and valleys, the broad plains and shallow crevices, as well as the long and short shapes in the body.

Working on the head allows you to feel what molding your hands is all about. With your partner lying on his back, place your hands on your partner's head. Rest your fingers along the side of your partner's skull, with your thumbs resting on his forehead. Let your hands rest, breathe softly, and instruct your receiver to relax. Refer to **FIGURE 12-1** to check your hand placement.

FIGURE 12-1

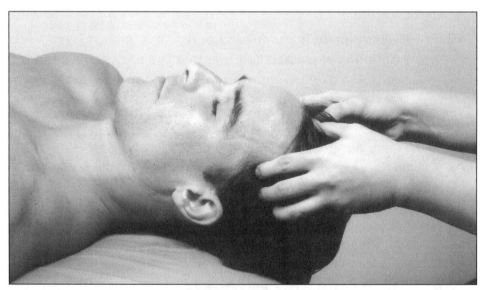

▲ Molding your hands to the head.

To use the petrissage technique, circle on the skin with one hand, pulling it up between your fingers and your thumb, and squeezing it as you circle around. Use both hands: one hand holds, squeezes, and pinches a section of flesh; the other hand picks up the next section, pinching and squeezing; then the first hand takes over the next section; and so on over the entire area you are working on.

Using Friction and Compression

Friction moves the skin over the muscle, creating a warm feeling on the skin. When your fingers encounter a tight area, circle down on that area with your fingers. If necessary, hold your partner's body steady with one hand as you circle in on the tight spot with your other hand. Tight neck muscles respond when you circle in with your thumb, holding on the affected area for a moment, as shown in **FIGURE 12-2**.

FIGURE 12-2

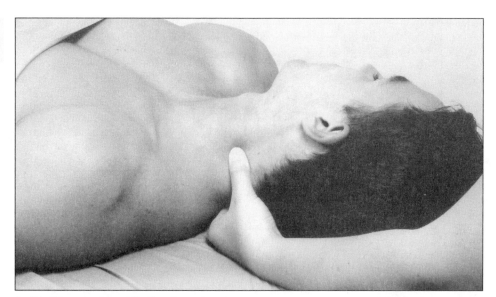

▲ Friction stroke with the thumb.

Compression brings a sense of wholeness within your body. Compression strokes are given with the flat palm of your hand while your fingers remain relaxed. You might press both palms on either side of the base of the spine, creating a human heating pad on the kidneys and adrenal glands. Or you might press using one palm on top of the other on the broad surface of your partner's back.

Using Stretching and Percussion

Stretching limbs helps to open the movement of the joints. An example of stretching is demonstrated in **FIGURE 12-3**, where the giver bends the receiver's leg toward his back, holding for a count of three before releasing. The receiver should lie passively to allow for easy stretching while the giver does this exercise.

FIGURE 12-3

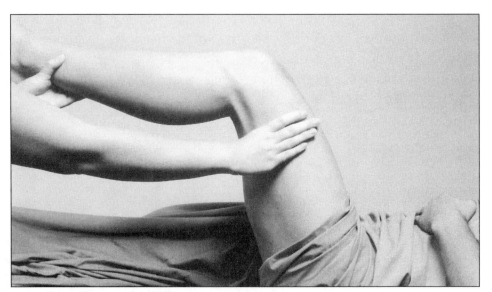

▲ Passive stretching of the leg.

There are many passive stretches you can do. Some others to try are:

- Bend each leg toward the chest and hold for a count of three; then release.
- Stretch each arm up over the head; rotate around and down.
- Gently stretch each arm back, opening up the chest.
- Gently stretch each leg up from the hip slowly, about ten inches off the floor.

Percussion is the tapping that often finishes a massage. Tapping is done with your fingertips or the sides of your hands in a karate-chop motion. Tap with your fingers down your partner's back, moving over the buttocks, and follow the legs to the ankles and down the soles. Using the sides of your hands, beat a staccato rhythm on your partner's back. Percussion puts the finishing touch as a complement to any massage.

Create Your Own Routine

There is no set routine for sensual massage. Your hands listen to the needs of the body beneath; you will feel the map of tension, stress, taut muscles, old pain, and tight joints. When you first place your hands on the back of your partner, close your eyes and see what information your hands receive. Imagine that you are involved in a dance and follow the lead of your partner. In fact, see what music your receiver would like to relax to and move your body with the rhythm of the beat.

Massage strokes are more effective when you move your body, and an instrumental piece with a soothing tempo allows you to move with ease. Set a pace and work your pattern with the music as your receiver relaxes. Your hands move to the music and your body becomes a fluid expression of the sound; you are involved in the sensual and intimate dance of massage. When it is your turn to be massaged, pick your music and relax as your giver moves with the flow.

Have fun inventing variations and improving different massages as you enjoy each other and the time together. There are many creative ideas that you can implement. Try one of the following options to get started:

- Give a massage in the tub using bath oil to work on the muscles of your partner.
- Find massage oil scented with your favorite flavor, such as strawberry or vanilla.
- Give a massage using only one or two strokes, not your favorites, and see what happens.
- Have a picnic and tuck massage oil in the basket so you can massage outdoors.
- Massage only the hands, or feet, or face, but spend at least twenty minutes on that one area.
- Show up at your partner's job and give a chair massage.

Communicate your thoughts and desires to your partner and be creative together. Take the time to invent intimate moments and enjoy exploring with each other. Massage is a form of loving communication that you can give and receive. Learning to relax and feel pleasurable touch is a gift you both can enjoy long after the experience. Ⓔ

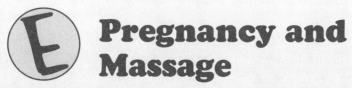

Chapter 13

Pregnancy and Massage

To be pregnant is miraculous; to find relief from the various discomforts that may accompany pregnancy is phenomenal. Massage during pregnancy is practiced in most cultures throughout the world. Massage provides relief from discomforts as well as support through the profound changes experienced during pregnancy. Massage is a tool of exchange that can be used by both expectant parents. Kind touch communicates love and acceptance and provides comfort and intimacy.

Why Prenatal Massage Is So Important

Pregnancy places a tremendous amount of pressure on the expectant mom's back, abdomen, shoulders, pelvis, legs, and feet, all of which must adapt to carrying the growing baby within. In addition, physiological changes create adverse stress for the mother-to-be as her arteries, veins, and lymph vessels increase their activity and hormones start pumping through her system.

The onset of pregnancy activates the secretion of the hormone relaxin. This hormone works to make the ligaments in the body looser and the joints more mobile. The joints and ligaments connecting the pelvic bones need to loosen, giving the pelvis the ability to stretch during the birth process. Relaxin is not discriminatory; therefore *all* the joints and ligaments in the body loosen during pregnancy. This may result in a variety of problems such as slipped vertebrae, joint and muscle pain, interrupted nerve supply to muscles, or uneven hip joints. In response to the loosening, muscles may tighten to support and stabilize the joints, resulting in muscle spasms.

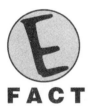

FACT

Relaxin begins to work the moment a woman becomes pregnant. The increase in flexibility of the pelvis, lower back, and hip joints helps make the delivery of the baby easier. Relaxin also helps to dilate the cervix during labor.

Benefits of Prenatal Massage

Prenatal massage works to relieve the stressors that pregnancy imposes upon the body by helping the woman take charge of herself, her body, and her experience in pregnancy. The relaxation provided with massage is profound. As you massage someone who is pregnant you help to lower her elevated heart and breath rate, creating a serene environment for the mother to be. Prenatal massage is beneficial in many aspects and creates an overall state of well-being. Some of the specific benefits of massage are that it can . . .

- Stabilize hormone levels.
- Increase overall circulation.
- Increase blood and oxygen supply.
- Stimulate lymphatic movement.
- Control varicose veins.
- Reduce swelling.
- Increase muscle tone.
- Relieve pressure from the back and shoulders.
- Promote nerve health.

Contraindications

Massage is essential in an uncomplicated pregnancy, but it can be harmful to certain pregnant women under certain circumstances. That is why it is very important for you to be sure any pregnant woman you plan to massage has gotten approval from her medical practitioner that massage is okay for her. There are specific conditions for which massage is not beneficial. Send a pregnant woman to her doctor if she tells you she has any of the following:

- High blood pressure
- Excessive swelling
- Toxemia
- Nausea or vomiting
- High fever
- Abdominal pain
- Vaginal bleeding

Massage During Labor

There are many signs that alert the expectant mother that she is approaching delivery of her child. Many women feel a sense of excitement and a surge of energy. Often this burst of energy is accompanied by behavior associated with an instinct known as nesting. The need to prepare the nest by cleaning the house and making last-minute adjustments to the nursery space are behaviors attributed to this instinct.

The expectant mom may experience deep lower back pain along with aching legs and pressure low in the pelvis. Her breasts may become more enlarged and heavier as the nourishing mother's milk increases in anticipation of the coming birth.

The Three Stages of Labor

Labor has three stages, each with very clear identifying features. The first stage starts when the cervix becomes thin and begins to open. There are very distinct contractions at this stage that serve to open the cervix wider in preparation for birth. Stage-one contractions can last for several hours, and usually last longer if this is a first baby.

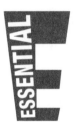

The opening of the cervix is known as dilation. In stage-one labor—the dilation stage—the cervix dilates to 7 cm., signaling the transition to stage two, the birth. Transition is complete when the cervix is dilated to 10 cm.

Staying mobile helps with stage-one labor. If the woman in labor can walk about she will speed up her labor and ride out the contractions more easily. During the early phase of stage-one labor, deep, slow breathing is helpful in dealing with the contractions. As contractions increase in intensity during the transition phase of stage one, breathing speeds up to a rapid panting as the woman works through each contraction.

The stage-two labor is the actual birth. Contractions come two to five minutes apart and the mother actively pushes during this period, bearing down with each contraction. After the baby is born, contractions continue until the placenta, or afterbirth, is expelled. The contractions following birth are stage-three labor, also known as the placental stage. These final contractions push out the placenta and constrict blood vessels that were torn during the delivery.

Massage in All Stages

Massage can be an important tool in every stage of labor. The reduction of pain is priceless, as is the lessening of anxiety. Massage brings relief from muscle contractions, helping at times to speed the birth. During the first stage of labor, loving touch through massage helps the laboring woman feel more confident and supported. As she moves into the transition phase, massage helps to reduce the anxiety during this heightened time of pain.

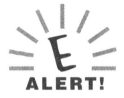

ALERT!

Massage can be a useful tool during labor if the woman in labor wishes to be touched. Always ask before attempting to administer massage to a woman who is in any stage of labor.

The giver of massage during labor provides a welcome oasis during a time that can feel isolating and out of control. Loving touch comforts and supports while creating a safe space. Caring touch helps the laboring woman to focus, giving her control of her body at a moment that seems without center. Massage gives strength and promotes endurance.

The placental stage is a wonderful time to give massage. The uterine contractions are still quite powerful, and you can assist in the delivery of the afterbirth by massaging the mother's belly. Steady rhythmic massage helps the mother expel the placenta so she may cuddle and rest with her baby. Massage is an essential tool in any labor room.

Following Birth

Massage is also helpful during the weeks of recovery following birth. This postpartum period is the time during which the woman's body returns to its normal prepregnancy state. Hormone levels even out and rebalance. As the hormonal balance is reestablished women often experience physical, emotional, and spiritual changes.

Postpartum Blues

Following birth, as the hormones work to retain balance, many women experience fatigue and the blues, which generally surface within ten days of the delivery. Postpartum emotions can surface as extreme highs and lows, mood swings that may seem irrational. Some women may seem irritable and anxious with no patience for anyone other than the baby. Tearfulness is a response to many situations during this period, and at times sadness may surface. Most women overcome the malaise by returning to a routine of proper rest and nutrition along with support from their community. Massage helps the mother to heal, too.

Some women experience postpartum depression, a far more severe consequence of the hormonal imbalance wreaking havoc in the new mother's body. This depression is more serious than the "baby blues." The woman suffering from postpartum depression undergoes mood swings, has difficulty concentrating, and may be anxious and irritable yet cannot express these emotions. Women who suffer with this depression feel unable to cope with their new infant; they feel powerless and inadequate. Anyone with these or similar symptoms should seek professional help. The use of compassionate touch through massage is a useful tool for additional support during this trying time.

Benefits of Massage After the Birth

A universal truth is that massage heals, and in cultures throughout the world massage is provided before, during, and after birth. After the birth, a new mother can massage her own belly to help with the production of lochia and the release of this discharge. Massage localized to the abdomen helps speed up the healing of the uterus and helps restore the elasticity of the skin. Massage of the lower back relieves tension. Overall, massage relieves muscle aches and pains and helps the mother regain energy and strength.

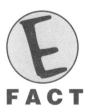

FACT

As the hormones return to balance, any excess hormones will leave the body as waste, resulting in a heavy volume of urine and excess perspiration. This release of toxins is accompanied by the production of lochia, a normal vaginal discharge that follows birthing. This discharge eventually disappears about two weeks after the birth.

Pregnancy Massage Essentials

Massage during all stages of pregnancy helps the expectant mother to maintain her health and sustain her energy level. Pregnancy is a joyous time when the body undergoes many changes as it provides protection and support for the baby.

Strokes for Pregnancy

The basic massage techniques you use on a pregnant woman are ones you have already learned, including effleurage, petrissage, tapotement, friction, and feathering. These include basic Swedish massage strokes as well as a few other techniques derived from Oriental bodywork. If you want to review some of these techniques, see Chapter 5.

Positioning the Receiver

The mother may feel pressure on the abdomen fairly soon into the term, so begin with the mother lying on her back, with a pillow under her knees for support. Her back should be flat on the surface you are working on. Some women may need more than one pillow under their knees and legs. A small pillow to support the neck may be all that is needed under her head early in the pregnancy. However, as the expectant woman moves toward full term, even lying on her back will become problematic. The growing baby within may press on the descending aorta and interfere with blood flow to the placenta.

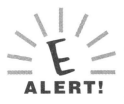

The aorta is the main artery supplying blood throughout the body. There are many branches that stem from the aorta. One of these branches, the descending aorta, is the branch that feeds the chest, the diaphragm, and the abdominal regions of the body. Too much pressure on it will interfere with the circulation through this artery.

Ultimately the pregnant woman feels best on her side, and the massage will need to be modified accordingly. However, for now, begin with the mother on her back if she is comfortable in that position.

A Simple Head and Neck Routine

Several components of the pregnancy massage routine are easy to perform on yourself, including the face and ear massage. This gives you a chance to practice your technique and become aware of how the receiver feels. It also gives you a chance to relax.

The Face

Use natural oil like jojoba oil and warm it in your hands before applying. Some people prefer cream on the face and others like nothing at all. Begin by applying gliding strokes up the neck and off the side of the jaw. Use both hands, one on each side of the face. Continue gliding onto the chin and up over the cheekbones. Glide up the forehead and off the head.

Return to the chin, still using both hands, and use light pinching to lift the flesh up along the jaw to behind the cheekbone. Continue to pinch and lift along the entire chin and cheekbone until the area is covered. Use very easy pinching strokes on the upper lip between the lip and the nose. Press with your index fingers on either side of the nose up to the forehead. Pinch along the ridge of the eyebrow from the outside of the face to the bridge of the nose; then pinch back from the ridge to the edge of the brow.

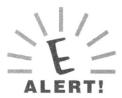
ALERT!

Massage affects the flow of fluid in the body. You do not want to push blood through a system that is experiencing a chemical or mechanical breakdown. In cases of extreme swelling, called edema, don't massage—you could make the situation worse.

Using all your fingertips, press from the top of the brow to the top of the forehead. Repeat this movement until the entire forehead has been worked. Now move up to the scalp and rub the entire head using a shampoo motion. At the base of the skull use your fingertips to hook under the two notches directly behind the ears. Gently press into the depression, and hold with your hands cupping the back of the head.

The Ears

Place your thumbs behind each ear, resting your thumb pads along the back of the ears; rest your index fingers on the sides of the cheeks in front of the ears. Gently stroke the edge of your index fingers along the entire surface of each ear. This will feel very soothing. Grasp each earlobe, with your thumbs on the back side and your index fingers pressing from the other side. Hold this position to a count of five.

Continue to work up along the edge of the ears, with your thumbs on the back side and your index fingers inside of each ear. Slightly pinch along the outside ridges of the ears. At the top of the ears, press your thumbs and index fingers together, and hold to a count of five. Bring your thumbs behind the fleshy lobes and rub your index fingers on the outsides of each lobe. Stroke down the entire lobes of both ears for two minutes; this will relax the whole body.

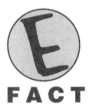

FACT

Working on the ears is actually a soothing reflexology technique that fits very well into massage. The reflexology points in the ear relax the spine and back as well as the internal organs. Stroking the lobe produces overall relaxation.

The Neck

Relax both your hands along the front of the woman's neck, gently stroking from the clavicle bones to the shoulders. Using both your hands gently glide from the base of the neck up to the chin, holding the chin in an easy stretch for the count of three. Carefully turn the head to one side and, using the fingers of both your hands, glide along the side of the neck up to the base of the skull. Repeat along this area using circular stretching strokes.

Turn the head to the other side and repeat the gliding and circling strokes. Move the head back to the center and place both hands under the base of the skull, cradling the head. Using all your fingers press, pull, and circle from the shoulder line up to the back of the skull, gently stretching at the head. Repeat this stroke at least three times. Lastly, stroke under the head with one hand following the other three times, finally letting the head rest.

Massaging the Body

Massage can relax the expectant mother, releasing muscle spasms and helping to reduce tension. As circulation is improved, the flow of blood and accompanying lymph drainage keeps the muscles and connective tissues healthy. Massage can tone tendons and ligaments, which helps keep joints flexible. Remember to use sufficient oil to keep your strokes smooth and gentle throughout the entire massage.

The Torso

Cover the woman's breasts with a towel, leaving the stomach uncovered, letting the cover drape everything below the stomach. Place the palms of both your hands flat on the chest just above the breasts, and press. This is a comforting compression move that releases built-up toxins. Now move to the right side of the mother, gently placing your hands on her stomach.

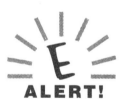

ALERT!

Never press hard on anyone's abdominal area, especially a pregnant woman's. In a pregnant woman, the organs move around as the baby grows, and the growing child is close to the surface of the abdomen. While massage is beneficial for the baby and the mother, any pressure must be gentle.

Move both your hands in a clockwise manner as you gently stroke with soft gliding motions over the entire abdominal area. Circle up to the ribs and down to the top of the pubic bone; circle up and back again. Always use slow, steady, and gentle strokes. The baby may respond to this loving touch.

The Arms

Move from the abdomen to the arms, working first one arm and then the other. With one hand on each side of the arm, wring down the arm and back up again, using this stroke to circulate the blood flow. Let both your hands glide down the arm from the shoulder to the hand. Repeat these gliding strokes three times. Hold the mother's hand in your hands, letting your fingers stretch the palm, pulling from the center as your thumbs rest on top of the hand.

Effleurage the inside of the arm from the wrist up to the underarm area and back to the wrist; repeat at least three times. Using both hands, petrissage down the arm from the shoulder to the wrist and back up; repeat twice. To complete this arm, use feather strokes from the shoulder to the wrist and back up to the shoulder; repeat three times. Move to the other arm and follow the same routine.

The Legs

Standing to the side of the mother, use both your hands to make long sweeping strokes up and down one leg. Sweep with a gliding effleurage stroke from the top of the foot up the front of the legs to the hip. Roll under the leg, and glide from the back of the thigh to the calf to the bottom of the foot. Your touch should be gentle and steady, with no deep pressure.

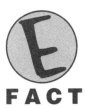
FACT

The weight gain a woman experiences during pregnancy is not only from the growth of the fetus. Amniotic fluid, which protects the baby from shock and regulates temperature, causes some of the weight gain, and so does the placenta, which feeds the growing baby and produces needed hormones.

Back at the ankle, use both hands and circle the pads of your fingers along either side of the shinbone up to the knee. Use a very easy, gentle touch at the knee, circling around the kneecap, but never pressing directly on it. Then, with both your hands, use your fingers to move up the underside of the calf from the ankle to the knee. From the topside of the knee, circle and press with friction up the front of the thigh to the hip with the fingers of both your hands. At the hip, circle in deeply following the shape of the hip bone on to the side of the buttock.

Now gently glide down to the ankle with both hands cupping the leg. At the ankle, effleurage up the entire leg to the hip and back down again. From the ankle, press up the leg, applying a steady pressure with your fingers moving up along the front of the leg, remembering to move easily over the knee area. Lift the leg slightly and pull straight back with an even, steady pull. Glide from the toes to the ankle with both hands.

Glide up and down the foot a number of times using your open hands. Press down toward the ankle; circle your fingers under to the sole, keeping your thumbs on top of the foot; and pull up along the sole to the toes with a steady and even pressure. Place your thumbs on top of the foot with your fingers on the sole and stretch the skin to the sides. Stretch and pull, using your thumbs and fingers to relax all the muscles of the foot. Finish by gently feathering up and down the entire leg before moving to the other leg.

The Back

The best way to work on the back of a pregnant woman is to turn her on her side and place a pillow between her legs. Allow her to turn sideways while you hold up the drape so she can move with privacy. Once she is comfortably lying on her side, position a pillow under her head and another between her legs. These pillows create an extra cushion to help take pressure off the joints. Some mothers need a pillow under their stomachs, too. Adjust the cover so only the mother's back is exposed.

Effleurage the entire back with both hands from the hip to the neck, moving with a steady even stroke, applying more pressure with each full stroke. Allow your hands to feel for areas of stress and tightness. Focus first on the shoulder area, where often you will find a great deal of congestion. Move your fingers in a steady circular motion following the muscles from either side of the spine to the shoulder area. Of course, the side the mother is lying on will miss some of the massage at this time.

Starting at the buttock area and moving up to the neck, use your palm to circle the entire area with smooth, deep pressure. Let your hand feel the skin underneath it as the skin responds to the release. Use your entire hand to press and push along the spine up to the neck and shoulders. Circle and press the neck and shoulder area, again feeling for a restriction. Repeat the circle strokes from buttocks to neck three times, feathering down the back at the end.

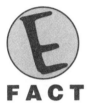

FACT

Friction helps to relieve tension in muscles and joints. As the constriction in the muscles is released you will see a red color in the area. This redness represents the increase in circulation as blood flows to the region that was congested.

Now circle and press on the hip and buttock with both hands; then, using your fingers, press in and hold in the fleshy area, the center of the hip, just below the hip bone. Knead the fleshy area, lifting and wringing, releasing the stress in the muscles there. With a pressing movement using your fingers, press along the side of the leg to the knee and back up to the hip. Place one hand on the shoulder and one hand on the hip, and press and hold at both places for the count of seven. Feather the entire area as you prepare to turn your receiver so that you can work on the other side.

Make sure to remove the pillows from between the legs and under the stomach. Again, hold the drape up to give the mother privacy as she turns to the other side. Repeat the entire back sequence.

You have just performed an easy routine for the pregnant woman. This massage or variations of this massage may be used throughout the entire pregnancy. During labor, if the mother permits, you can modify this routine, perhaps working only the back. After labor and during post-partum recovery, massage is a wonderful tool that will expedite the mother's healing. Massage between mother and father is an expression of love and compassion that can be shared from the beginning of pregnancy and throughout their lives. Celebrate touching with compassion. Incorporate massage as an essential tool in your daily life.

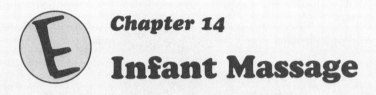

Chapter 14

Infant Massage

The importance of touch for a newborn is immeasurable. As the infant enters the world, the safe, warm, protected environment that has enveloped the baby during gestation is stripped away. Now baby is exposed to the stress of bright lights, loud noises, and open space. Massage is a tool that will help the newborn adapt to stress in a healthful, integrative manner. As stress is part of the cycle of learning, so is relaxation.

The Philosophy of Infant Massage

Infant and parent bonding is essential for proper development of the child. Massage encourages this bonding by forging the link between parents and their infant, providing a powerful supportive foundation. Proper development and growth are intrinsic to the infant's ability to process sensory, motor, and cognitive input. Constant touching, talking, cuddling, and stroking of an infant promotes healthy growth and provides positive stimulation for mental and emotional well-being.

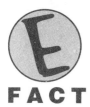

FACT

Touched infants are less irritable and better able to sleep. Emotionally the infant who is massaged has a more even nature, cries less, and interacts more with her parents. The infant's reaction to the stimulus of touch encourages increased motor ability and a greater degree of mental alertness.

Newborns receive many signals as they attempt to cope with life outside the uterus. The skin represents the first form of communication— as the infant is welcomed into the world the initial stimulus is presented through touch. During a typical labor, the contractions of the uterus that thrust the baby forward also stimulate the systems of the infant's body, preparing the baby to function outside of the mother. In essence, labor contractions massage the baby, getting all systems ready to function once the baby is born.

The Necessity of Touch

Touch is imperative from the moment of birth and is a requirement for the continued health and development of the newborn. The more often the newborn is touched, caressed, held, exercised, bathed, and stimulated through any form of loving touch, the better the progression of development for the infant. During the first year of life babies cannot be touched enough. Touch transmits love and safety to the infant, allowing for enhanced growth as well as proper functioning as the baby grows.

Touch Is a Two-Way Street

The bonding between parents and their infant is essential for all involved, and touch promotes this bond. Parents receive as much by giving soothing touch as the baby who receives it. The love and enjoyment transmitted by touch is unequaled. Loving touch reinforces the importance of the developing relationship between mature adults and their infant.

Siblings and their newborn family member need to bond as well. Involving a sibling in appropriate care of an infant develops a loving, responsible relationship early on. Include your older child in the massage of the new baby, with supervision of course. As the older child gives to the younger, a special sibling bond appears, and massage helps to form this close-knit tie early on. As siblings massage the newborn they also receive. The satisfaction of bonding with the baby and other involved family members supports the development of self-esteem and love throughout the entire family.

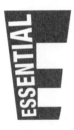

Depending upon the age of the siblings, they can be involved in many bonding activities. Older children love to hold, cuddle, hug, and kiss the baby. Assisting in bath time is another bonding tool that is fun for the sibling.

The Effects of Massage on Infants

If you lovingly touch your newborn frequently you are encouraging strength, intelligence, depth, and emotional security, and you are supporting physiological growth. A baby who is massaged is alert and responsive. This infant quickly develops adaptation techniques to his constantly changing and stimulating environment. Contact is the comfort infants crave the most; an infant without nurturing care will not thrive or, at best, will develop poorly. Gentle massage supports the nervous system, allowing the baby to develop a strong immune system as well as good neurological development. Also, a baby's tiny muscles make up only one fourth of the baby's weight, and massage helps those muscles grow. Babies who are massaged are healthier with less evidence of colds, infections, and digestive upsets.

Relaxation for Easy Breathing

While infants develop within their mothers they receive oxygen from the placenta. Upon birth the newborn must adapt immediately to breathing without help. Touch becomes an essential ingredient in helping the infant to relax, while the infant learns to breathe deeply on his own. The mother will instinctively hug, kiss, caress, and rock her newborn and constantly rub her baby's back and chest. This massaging assists in the further development of the respiratory system as well as the transition from shallow to deep breathing.

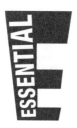

Adequate rocking by the mother or other caregiver creates an environment that is reassuring to the baby. Rocking feels like the mother's womb and supports calmness within the baby. Research has shown that touching in the form of rocking and massaging helps to prevent sudden infant death syndrome (SIDS).

Production of Hormones

Massage supports the endocrine system, which produces hormones that dictate the function of the various organs within the body. The activity of every organ is fueled in part by these hormones. Good touch enables the hormone-producing glands of the endocrine system to function in a state of balance, or homeostasis. Infants who receive massage have greater hormonal support, which in turn increases the activity of their vital organs. Remember, a baby's organs are still learning how to function on the outside of the womb, so stimulation on a hormonal level is good.

Support of the Nervous System

The central nervous system—the brain and the spinal cord—works with the endocrine system to support homeostasis. Massage assists the central nervous system by encouraging the formation of nerve and brain cells, including the myelin sheath that protects nerve fiber and serves to speed nerve impulses from the brain to other parts of the body. The myelin sheath is not completely formed before the baby is born, but it responds rapidly to tactile stimulation. During infancy this formation of cells and myelin is very important, and massage contributes to the growth and support of an infant's nerve health.

Relief from Stress and Overstimulation

Being born is stressful, as is surviving outside of the womb. Massaging the newborn and the growing infant helps the baby adapt to the physical world. Entering into the unknown is scary and confusing on any level, but imagine the feelings of a newborn. Massage helps the baby relax from what would otherwise be overstimulation. Touch is essential for the baby to live a healthy life. There is no such thing as too much loving touch.

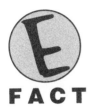

FACT

A baby receives sensory input while in the womb, but the baby's awareness begins upon entry into the physical realm. Everything the baby is exposed to represents a stimulus. As the baby learns to use his or her sensory organs to interpret these stimuli, all the baby's senses contribute to healthy growth and development.

Stress introduces the opportunity to adjust, to take the new and unknown and make it familiar. However, a baby who has only the constant input of strange and new situations and no reassuring touch may tire and burn out. Massage helps an infant cope and adapt. It gives the baby the time to relax and recharge, enabling the infant to continue to grow. If you introduce massage early in a child's development, he will be better equipped to deal with the stress of life as he grows up.

Techniques for Infant Massage

You use some of the same familiar strokes you learned for adults on babies, too, but your strokes on infants are not as deep as those you use on adults. The initial touch you use on adults is now called "familiar touch" when you address the infant's body at the beginning of a session. Infants love to be touched and they respond to light, gentle touch once they become familiar with the sensation. You want the baby to become accustomed to massage, not to feel surprised or threatened. The loving massage that you give will bond your relationship in a wonderful way.

The touch that you apply should be light yet firm. Work slowly and easily, keeping contact with the baby through your touch, your voice, and your eyes. Choose a natural unscented, light oil or cream to work on your baby, staying away from essential oils and oils derived from nuts.

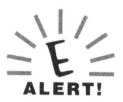

ALERT!

Essential oils are like medicine. A trained aromatherapist must be consulted before using aromatherapy oils on anyone because people can have allergic reactions to them. Nut oils can also produce serious allergenic responses. If you decide to use any of these products, always test them on a small patch of skin first.

Using Familiar Touch

This touch is the first stroke you will apply. It is a gentle stroke that is more of a holding move, using one or both of your hands, depending upon the size of your hands and the baby. Without removing clothes, gently stroke down the baby's front and then back. This is a feathering technique using your fingertips; the touch is light and steady. You will touch the baby from head to toe, talking softly, explaining perhaps what you are doing. This touch will help the infant become familiar with the concept of extended touch. Gently rest your hands on the baby's belly before turning over to do the back.

Using Effleurage and Petrissage

Once the baby has become accustomed to routine touch, you may begin to effleurage. These long gliding strokes work well on the torso and extremities. With both hands, use your entire palms and the flats of your fingers to apply a light yet firm pressure over the baby's body, stroking down and up.

You will not be kneading the baby's back. However, the baby's arms and legs usually respond well to wringing, milking, rolling, and squeezing. Wringing is twisting and squeezing the arms or legs from the bottom to the top. Do it gently and fluidly. Milking is exactly as it sounds: One hand follows your other as you gently milk from the baby's foot or hand to the baby's hip or shoulder. Rolling is placing the baby's arm or leg between your hands as you actually roll it between them.

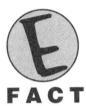

FACT

Infant massage can begin from the moment you hold your baby with soft easy strokes along your baby's covered back, as your newborn cuddles on your chest. The sooner you touch your newborn the sooner your baby feels secure, loved, and relaxed. Massaging your infant supports the development of your relationship with your child.

Using Circling

This stroke is applied with a slight amount of pressure from your fingertips or palms as they move in small circles. Circling is often applied along the sides of the spine, on the buttocks, around the hips, and on the abdomen. Circling brings you into an area and out again in a continual applied rhythm.

Using Stretching and Pressing

Stretching helps the baby develop a greater range of motion. Newborns are still mimicking their posture in the womb, so easy stretching gives the baby an alternative position to strive for. Gently stretch the baby's limbs into an open position, pulling only as far as the baby will open. You can also stretch the skin by pressing down with your fingers and slightly stretching it away by pulling your fingers to either side. These strokes are good to use as transitions or ending techniques.

A Simple Routine

To perform the massage you can hold the baby on your knees, or you can place the baby on a pad on the floor or in the crib, whichever is most comfortable for both of you. Choose a space that allows you to keep your back straight while you move your body in rhythm with your strokes. Make sure the room is warm. Your oil should be room temperature, but you should also warm it a bit between your hands before you apply it. Your hands should be clean, your nails trimmed, and your jewelry removed. Undress your baby and wrap him in a towel.

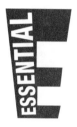

Wherever you massage the baby, create a quiet space for you and the infant. The TV and radio are best turned off, and if you play music choose a relaxing tape with gentle sounds. Arrange for massage time to be quiet playtime for any siblings, too.

Try to establish a regular routine with your infant. Give your baby time to digest his food, but make sure your baby is comfortable so he does not need to eat while you are in the middle of a massage.

Begin with the Legs and Feet

Babies love to have their feet and legs touched so this is a good area to begin. Lay your baby face up with his feet near you. Talk to your infant, explaining what you are doing as you unfold the towel from around him. Use a small amount of oil, just enough to allow your hands to glide on your baby's legs. Hold the right foot with your left hand and gently stroke up the leg from the ankle to the thigh and back down again, repeating three times. Place your hand under the leg and glide up and back on the underside three times.

Grasp the baby's ankle gently, lift the leg, and use a milking stroke from the ankle to the thigh and back again. Switch hands and, with the same milking stroke, work the thigh to the hip and buttock and back to the ankle again. If your baby likes this stroke, do it again. If the infant seems fidgety complete only one cycle. The baby will become more accustomed to this stroke the more often you massage your infant.

Now bring both your hands to one side of the baby's right leg. Beginning at the ankle, use a wringing motion, moving each hand in the opposite direction as you wring up the leg to the thigh and back down again. Repeat. As you twist back and forth be gentle—this is a wringing, not a friction, movement. Lift the leg up and wring to the thigh and gently effleurage down to the foot.

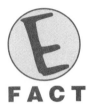

FACT

The foot is one of the best places to massage on an infant. In fact, you could just massage the feet and the baby would relax. Notice how calm the baby becomes as you hold the right foot in your hands and gently stretch the sole of the foot with your thumbs.

With your fingers resting on the top of the foot, let your thumbs meet at center of the bottom of the foot. Stretch the skin out to the sides and back again. Continue this stretching down the entire surface to the heel.

Cup the foot between both your hands and gently wring the foot, up and down. Using your thumbs make gentle circles around the ankle and circle onto the top of the foot. Slowly squeeze each toe very gently and then press your thumbs into the ball of the foot. Let your thumbs make walking movements along the ball of the foot. Rest both your hands on the foot, feeling the heat from your palms permeate in the foot. Repeat this sequence on the left leg and foot, starting with the wringing motion from the ankle to the thigh.

Next, bend each leg by holding the foot at the ankle and bending the knee. Gently stretch out each leg and bend it again. Begin to press and stretch the legs at opposite times as though the baby is riding a bicycle. Now bend both legs at the same time and stretch those legs out once more. Gently roll each leg between your hands from the ankle to the hip and back again.

Chest and Abdomen

The natural progression from the legs is to move up to the abdomen and chest region. Massaging the abdomen helps with digestion and elimination; massaging the chest helps stimulate the lungs and the heart.

The baby should be more relaxed now, especially if you have continued to talk quietly, letting him know what you are doing.

Begin with a gentle press on your baby's belly, turning this press into a circle that moves from the right to the left. Continue circling clockwise on your baby's stomach with steady, gentle movements.

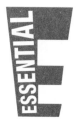

Failure to thrive is an infant's inability to grow and flourish. Traditionally this condition was linked to inadequate pituitary production, especially the growth hormone. Later studies proved that the insufficient hormone production from the pituitary gland is caused by the lack of parental love. Massage is one of the tools used to correct this lack.

Use your fingers and gently trace the outline of this circle from the right side of the abdomen up to the waist, across the belly, and down the left side. Continue to make slow, deliberate kneading strokes inside this circle, following in the same clockwise direction. The pressure here is still gentle but steady as you move around the area of the colon and small intestines. Eventually you will end up at the belly button, where you press gently and hold for the count of five.

Place both your hands on the baby's chest, with your palms on the belly and your fingers resting on the rib cage. This is a very comforting position because the pressure from your warm, loving hands gives the baby a feeling of security. Gently press your hands out to the baby's sides, stretching and pressing as you move. Finally, circle down the sides to the belly and back up the center to the chest again. Repeat.

Hands and Arms

Effleurage down the chest and up again as you move your hands across the baby's shoulders and down the arms. Bring both hands back to the shoulders and glide down both arms to the fingers. Repeat this stroke again, gently stretching the baby's arms out straight. You may glide and stretch two or three times as you are opening the baby's arms with this move.

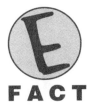

FACT

If your baby pulls away and wraps her arms close to her chest, do not force the arms apart or away from this protective stance. Some babies do not like having their arms massaged. Simply massage the baby's arms in this hugging posture. As the baby becomes more familiar with the touch, she will open her arms.

Now lift the right arm and milk from the hand to the underarm area. Gently stroke with your fingers under the arm, moving your fingers toward the heart. Squeeze and twist in a wringing stroke up the arm and down; repeat. Lightly stroke down both sides of the arm to the fingers and gently open the hand. Next, stroke with your fingertips on the inside of the baby's hand as you rest the hand in your other palm. Use your thumb and index finger to press each tiny finger, gently. Do not pull the fingers! Make small circles around both sides of the baby's wrist before you finish by stroking the top of the hand. Repeat this process on the other arm.

The Back

Place your baby on his stomach with his legs stretched toward you. He may be on a flat surface or across your legs—whichever both of you are comfortable with. Use a soft effleurage stroke, moving down the back, over the buttocks, and up the back again. Place your hands horizontally across the baby's back, one hand leading the other. Use a soft effleurage stroke and gently glide down the back, over the buttocks, and up to the neck several times.

Place both hands on the back with your fingers facing the shoulders. Glide up to the shoulders, along the side of the neck and down the backs of the arms. Repeat this stroke. Now place both hands on the back and stroke with the entire hand down the back to the heels, using firm light pressure. Repeat.

Bring both hands onto the back and circle with your fingertips over the entire back area. Then gently knead the buttocks with the palms of your hands in small circles. Stroke each of your hands down the leg to the heel, gently holding the heels. Finish with soft feather touches, staying in contact with your baby while you softly stroke from the neck to the feet. Place both hands on the back and rest.

The Face

Turn the baby face up, resting both your hands ever so lightly on your baby's head as you look into his eyes and talk to him. Softly stroke down the sides of the skull to the jaw, bringing your fingers to the chin. If your baby likes this movement repeat it two or three times. Play peekaboo by placing your open hands lightly over your baby's face. Then use your fingers to stretch the skin softly across the forehead. Gently circle with your fingertips along the sides of the forehead.

Using your thumbs and index fingers pinch along the jaw up to the cheekbones. Place your thumbs on either side of the nose and stroke up along the side of the nose and out across the cheekbones. Stroke across the cheekbones and up to the ears, letting your fingers brush lightly on the ears. Place your thumbs on the inside of the ear lobes and your index fingers on the fleshy outside. Easily and lightly stroke down the lobes, squeezing them between your thumbs and index fingers. Stroke down the earlobes several times, and watch how relaxed the baby becomes.

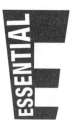

The earlobe is a point used in reflexology and other pressure methods for relaxation. All babies know this innately—a baby will stroke her ear when she is tired and needs comfort. The gentle stroking of the lobe triggers the nervous system to release chemicals that help relax the body.

Stretches

The best way to finish the massage is to perform some easy stretches with your baby. The infant is already lying face up, so hold the baby's hands in your hands and stretch the arms across the chest, and then open them. Continue to bring the arms in and across, and open, perhaps singing or talking as you make exercise play. Carefully stretch the arms up over the head, out to the sides, and then down, essentially moving in a semicircle.

Next, hold your baby's ankles in your hands and stretch one leg over the other across the abdomen, repeating several times. Now gently stretch the legs down away from the torso in a straight line before pushing the legs up to a bent-knee position. Repeat this move twice, making sure your baby is enjoying the stretching. Using gentle effleurage, stroke across your baby's body from shoulder to hip, continuing down the leg and off the foot. Press your hands easily into your baby's chest and hold. Thank your baby for a wonderful experience.

Massage and the Older Child

Once you have established a massage routine with your baby it is easy to continue with this as he grows. Loving touch becomes a special part of your baby's day whether it is enjoyed after a bath or as part of a diaper-change or bedtime routine. All babies need comfort and care throughout the first two years of life. From the moment they wake up to the ritual at sleep time, loving, comforting touch is crucial to your child's health and well-being.

From infant through toddler to older child, everyone benefits from massage. Massage can help the older child to relax not only muscles but feelings as well.

Communicating Through Loving Touch

If you want to find out how your older child is feeling, provide a safe comfort zone through massage. This is a zone where the child can share feelings. Older children have fears that they often do not know how to express. They may harbor resentment, anger, worry, fear, or a sense of abandonment. Loving touch creates the safe space needed to let out those fears and release of tension.

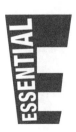

Massage is a form of holding, and until puberty children need to be stroked and held by their parents. "I love you" is best said through touch until the child reaches about the age of twelve. Children believe what they can touch and what they can feel.

Modifying the Infant Massage Routine

You have established a massage routine with your newborn that you can change to fit your growing child. All the massage strokes you used when your child was an infant still apply, but now they must cover a larger area because your child's limbs and torso have grown. So you must adjust your movements to compensate. When you glide use a more sweeping technique to carry you along the longer limbs. The circles can be larger, too, but the pressure is still gentle. Your child is old enough to give you feedback, so be sure to ask what feels good and what does not.

Teach your child to circle on his abdomen, which will help him to get rid of tension in the stomach and help with elimination. Now that the child is older, teach him a stretching routine the child can do whenever he likes. Exercise together as you reach for the sky and bend to the ground. Stretch your arms out to the side and bend sideways; then stand tall and twist. Stand on one foot as you bend your other leg at the knee, lifting the foot off the floor, learning to balance. Lie on the floor together with knees bent and make bicycle movements, pushing first one leg and then the other. Each of you hug yourselves, stretching your folded arms up to your chin and back to your chest.

Finish by teaching your child to stroke his own earlobes. Show him how to gently stroke along the lobe with the index finger, supporting with the thumb.

From birth through childhood, massage can be used to promote healthy emotional and physical growth. Start early, and encourage everyone in your family to become involved with the loving gift of massage.

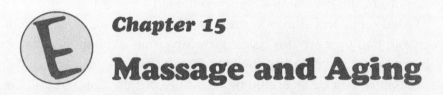

Chapter 15

Massage and Aging

One thing you can absolutely count on is that you, along with the rest of us, will grow old. Today you are one day older than you were yesterday. Aging is a visible biological fact. The design of the body supports the concept of aging and we can embrace healthy choices that allow us to age youthfully. Take care of your body and you will remain vital and fit, with the energy to embark on many exciting new journeys.

The Principles of Elder Massage

Aging is part of our life as we progress through life's many stages. To reach the status of an elder is an accomplishment. To be healthy and strong as an elder is triumphant. Massage, along with other supportive health measures, greatly increases our ability to grow old and stay young. Preventive health programs support continued homeostasis.

Based on information from the U.S. Census Bureau, people eighty-five years old and over are the fastest growing group of people in the country. While many of the elderly population are active and healthy, maintaining their independence longer, the oldest of the old do begin to fail. People older than eighty-five may face a decline in health as well as loss of independence and loss of their partners. More women than men reach the oldest age group, so many elderly women are living alone without partners, which can turn into isolation, which is an increasing threat to the elderly. Massage is a way to combat this threat.

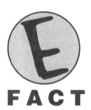

FACT

According to the Population Resource Center, there are approximately thirty-four million people in the United States today over age sixty-five. This represents 13 percent of the total population. About one in eight people living today are considered to have reached the age of retirement. By the year 2020 this number will have increased to one in five people.

The Social Connection

Massage for the elderly not only provides physical healing, it also provides the opportunity to interact with someone else, lifting them out of their isolation. Folks who are confined, whether through physical limitations or living arrangements, benefit from the time spent with another person before, during, and after a massage. Before a massage the receiver generally shares any physical concerns that she may be experiencing at the time. During the massage the recipient may feel more relaxed, more in touch with her body, and certainly more alive. After a massage the communication gates are fully open as the receiver basks in the enjoyment of caring touch and loving concern.

The Effects of Massage on the Elderly

Touch is important during any phase of life, as expressed by Ashley Montagu, the late pioneer and revered expert in the field of touch, who wrote: "It is especially in the aging that we see touching at its best as an act of spiritual grace and a continuing human sacrament." With the loss of so many senses and functions as one ages, the need for healing touch is crucial. Our elder community needs, wants, and deserves the compassionate touch that massage can provide.

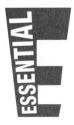

Too often the concept of aging brings to mind isolation, illness, and death. You can help an elder stay in touch with not only the exciting aspects of growing older but the joy of being touched. Massage for the elder population is important for their emotional, physical, mental, and spiritual well-being.

With aging, the elasticity of the skin is affected. Wrinkles and spotting often appear, along with dryness and a change in pigment. As people age their receptors for touch become less sensitive, especially the nerve endings in their palms. Informed touch stimulates the skin and helps keep it supple and alive, while at the same time reinforcing the tone of the muscles that lie under the connective tissue providing support.

Some of the benefits of massage that particularly affect the elderly include these:

- Stimulates the appetite
- Releases hormones
- Improves sleep
- Reduces joint pain
- Relieves swelling
- Stimulates circulation
- Lowers blood pressure
- Supports elimination

Massage is helpful for virtually all of the needs an elder has.

Seniors Give Back

Many of those who have lived a long life appreciate and understand how giving is receiving. To age is to blossom, and elders are the sweet bloom from the buds of youth. Many seniors continue to appreciate the taste of life and the flow of the dance as they sway to the rhythm that beats for them. Who better understands the need to touch another human with compassion and respect than someone who has lived a long life in the company of others?

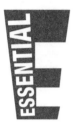

When you were a child your mom would hold you and stroke you and make your hurts go away. Your dad may have held your hand until you were too old and you said out loud you didn't like it, but secretly you felt loved and protected. Touch allows you to relate how much you care without the use of the spoken word.

Studies have shown that elders do feel just as good giving a massage as receiving one. Giving a massage says "I care enough to find out about you." When a younger member of the family receives a massage from Grandmother or Grandfather, the message is "you are important to me." Often children do not perceive the elders in the family as connecting with them in a real and meaningful way. So teach yourself to give a massage to your grandchildren or other loved ones. Organize your group of friends and have a massage party, or learn self-massage. Loving contact is for everyone, and massage is a special time together that allows communication on many levels.

When Massage Is Okay

Massage and aging for the most part are complementary. Massage can discourage the rapid onset of illness and aging by helping the elderly to remain strong. Working on the muscles of an older person helps that person to have more control of her or his body; the recipient becomes less stiff and has fewer aches and pains. Better muscle control leads to better coordination and dexterity, which both tend to suffer with age. Many people seem to forget that touch is therapeutic. Whatever stage of life you are in, massage has a place in your wellness program.

When Massage Is Not Okay

Today doctors and other health providers accept and applaud the concept of compassionate touch on all populations, especially the elderly, but it is always important to make sure the doctor knows about any additional health measures a patient is taking, including massage. Although the benefits of massage are plentiful, there are certain medical conditions that signal caution against massaging an elder. The conditions that contraindicate massage are:

- Severe swelling
- Open sores
- Bruises
- Inflammation
- Extreme sensitivity
- Blood clot
- Varicose veins

If an elder suffers from any of these conditions, a full-body massage is not appropriate. If none of the conditions indicated are near the face, a gentle face massage may be considered, with a medical practitioner's consent. Easy gliding strokes from the neck up to the forehead will provide comfort and the elder will benefit from the attention. If it is impossible to give a massage, simply holding hands provides a caring touch full of compassion and will be appreciated.

There are other conditions that require the approval of the receiver's medical practitioner. These are:

- Undergoing chemotherapy
- Undergoing radiation therapy
- Recovering from surgery

- Recovering from a stroke
- Recovering from a heart attack
- Living with osteoarthritis

Again, kind touch is healing touch and any form of touching is better than not touching at all. A hand that is held or patted combined with a hug, while not a massage, still provides caring support.

Techniques and Considerations for Elder Massage

Most of the techniques that you have learned so far are appropriate for massage on an elder. The massage strokes of effleurage, petrissage, pressing, and tapotement are all effective when working with the elderly population.

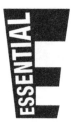

Inside the aging body is a young person, someone who feels that his body seems to have forgotten how to play. Exercise, proper diet, and continued bodywork are part of a lifestyle that allows a person to live life in a continuum rather than feel betrayed as the body fails.

Preparing for an Elder Massage

Elders can chill easily, so remain mindful of this and keep a light blanket close by. Some folks may not be able to climb onto a table or lie on a floor mat. Adapt accordingly, perhaps sitting your elderly recipient sideways on a chair or on a stool pushed up to the bed so the recipient can lean her head on the soft surface. Take your time and improvise with your space until you find what works.

Remember that many members of the senior population move at a slower pace than you do. Use this time to connect with the recipient as she moves slowly to the workspace, and continue your connection afterwards when the recipient slowly puts on her shoes. Understand that this is your lesson in patience and learning to wait. Breathe in the moment and enjoy your relationship with the receiver. What a gift to be allowed to slow down and enjoy.

Personalized Contact

Throw away any preconceived stereotypical notions you might have, and greet each senior as an individual with his or her own strengths and frailties. Honor the differences of every person you deal with, regardless of age. There may be certain issues that everyone in the older age group have in common, but remember, everyone is also different!

Understand that not all seniors are frail; many still have strong muscles under their visually aging skin. All people hold tension in their body regardless of physical strength. The knots and tightness you find in others may be present with an elder too. Thin elderly bodies do not necessarily mean weak, brittle bodies. Yes, the bones of elderly people are certainly more brittle and their joints are less flexible than those of younger people, but treat every person as an individual and assume nothing.

Setting Boundaries

Often elders live alone, without many visitors, and no set schedule. Often the highlight of the day is a visit from someone like you who is going to spend quality time with them. By providing a massage and an experience of companionship, you are brightening an elderly person's day. You, on the other hand, may have a full schedule, and this stop is only a part of your busy day. This is where clarity and good communication are important.

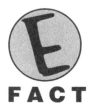
FACT

The MacArthur Foundation study on aging inspired Dr. Robert Kahn to cowrite *Successful Aging* (Pantheon Books, 1998), where he states that "We are hard-wired to live in interdependent groups, whether those groups be families, clans, or nations." Aging people still require family and friends, and without these connections the elderly will have a difficult time surviving.

Be very clear on the amount of time you intend to spend on this visit, keeping in mind that you will, indeed, need more time with the elderly, so plan for it. When you work with an elder the actual time you spend on the massage may be less than the time you work on younger people. However, your elder receiver needs extra time to prepare, to receive, and to recover. In addition, the older person will want to share the interesting points of his or her life—things that happened recently and things from the past. Give yourself enough time to enjoy the visit, give a quality massage, and still be able to leave when you planned.

A Routine for Senior Massage

Your routine will change according to the person you are working on. However, you can design a blueprint that you may adjust as needed. Consider styling a shorter session, at least initially. Be aware that an elderly person may not be able to lie in one position for too long at a time. And you may need to provide extra support with certain positions. Also ask how much clothing the receiver wishes to keep on, if any. Some people, no matter what age, prefer to receive massage through the cover, while others feel very comfortable completely in the buff. Use oil that is easily absorbed by the skin and remember to ask whether your massage partner prefers scented or not. Finally, make sure the temperature in the room is comfortable for the receiver.

Back and Shoulder Massage

If the receiver decides that she would like you to work the back and shoulders, and she can lie facedown for a short period of time, help her into a position that works best for her. Place pillows in areas that need extra support, and cover the recipient with a flannel sheet. Make the receiver as comfortable as possible, and remember to check in to see if she needs to move. Often a short time spent working on the back is as much as your elder recipient can tolerate in that position.

Rest both your hands on the receiver's covered back for a moment.

Then pull back the cover, tuck it around the waist, and apply oil with a gentle but firm effleurage stroke on the back, feeling for tension as you glide from the waist to the shoulders and back again. Your hands and fingers will tell you where to hold and press after you finish applying the oil. Glide along the shoulders and the backs of the arms, moving with a steady, even rhythm.

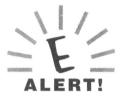

ALERT!

If your receiver is experiencing muscle spasms do not massage that area. A muscle spasm is a quick, involuntary contraction often due to the irritation of the nerves that assist the muscle. Use another form of relaxation, such as reflexology or Reiki, until the spasms have been corrected.

Return to the areas of tension and gently petrissage between the shoulder blades and around the neck. Remember to use steady, even pressure without digging, and be aware of any fragile areas. Constantly check with the receiver to make sure your pressure is fine. You may be surprised to learn the receiver wants you to press more firmly. Knead along the shoulders and then glide over the entire area again.

Moving On to the Arms and Legs

Remove any pillows or bolsters from under the legs before helping your receiver turn over onto her back. Be supportive; you may have to gently help the recipient up while keeping the drape tucked in for privacy. Carefully assist in any way your receiver needs and then help her to reposition.

Once the supports are back under the legs and perhaps under the neck and shoulders, too, effleurage one leg with both your hands. Use firm gliding strokes from the ankle to the knee and then from the knee to the hip. Repeat at least twice before gently kneading the hip area. Again let your fingers be your eyes as you feel where the tension is, while listening to the receiver as well. Glide again over the entire leg and repeat the sequence on the other leg.

Work the arms with the same strokes. Start with one arm and effleurage with both your hands from the wrist to the elbow and then from the elbow to the shoulder, using firm gliding movements. Repeat on the other arm. Remember to stroke the joints with a feathering movement. Do not apply pressure. Then knead in the shoulder areas with both hands, using extra caution as you approach the neck. Do not apply any massage to the center of the neck as this area is contraindicated. Gently feather off the shoulders and move to the head.

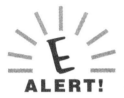

ALERT!

Pay attention to the person you are working on as you continue to stay in touch, assessing if the receiver needs to turn or get up. Alter your techniques to fit the body you are working on, and become aware of any limitations.

Strokes for the Face and Head

Stand behind the receiver and gently stroke up the face with both hands. Move from the chin, over the cheeks, and pull off at the forehead. Use circular kneading movements over the entire face, always moving up toward the forehead. Circle your fingers in at the jaw, easing tension that may accumulate in that region. Use feather strokes up the chest, along the sides of the neck, and over the face. Rest your hands, palms flat, over the eyes and hold still.

Using shampoo strokes work the entire top and back of the head, gently lifting the head so you can work the back of the scalp. Rest the head in your hands with your fingertips gently pressing in at the base of the skull. Hold here and breathe. Ask your receiver to breathe with you, slowly and gently.

Carefully remove your hands, check to make sure the recipient is fine, and go wash your hands. This gives the receiver time to relax and rest. When you return help the receiver off the table. Remember that elders tend to move a bit slower, so pace your movements with the receiver's. Remember to include some social time at the end of the massage, because talking with the elderly is just as important as your touch.

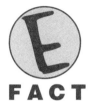

FACT

As you age you may find that you feel and function differently. You may feel stiff in the morning, taking a bit more time to begin your day. You can choose to make the most of this by making this the time to practice some of the relaxation exercises or self-massage techniques you have learned. This will help you work through the stiffness that your muscles and joints may be experiencing.

Touch and Dying

You will find that many people do not want to spend time with someone who is in the process of transition to death, because this means confronting their own fear of dying. This is a time when a dying person needs others the most, and if you can overcome your own fears you can provide a powerful gift. Understand that this person needs your sensitivity, your willingness to serve, and your compassionate touch. There are no set rules or regulations here other than to proceed with honor and respect, being mindful of the comfort of the person. Trust that your heart will guide you, and you will be appropriate. Be sensitive to the condition of the person, understanding that change is the constant state of affairs in which this person lives. The wants and needs of the person in transition can fluctuate from moment to moment.

You can help the person deal with the emotional stress of the situation as well as the physical discomfort. Approach with love and honesty, giving what you can. Know that compassionate, loving touch is essential during this time, whether it is a foot rub, a shoulder rub, or holding hands.

You are a teacher and a student, giving and receiving simultaneously. The intention to help on any level ensures that you are providing what is needed at any given time. The giving of kind touch breaks down all barriers while the sharing of this touch is splendid.

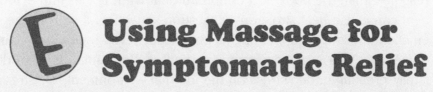

Chapter 16

E Using Massage for Symptomatic Relief

Homeostasis is the internal balance of the body's systems, and stress is the stimulus that upsets that balance. Both physical and psychological stress can upset homeostasis. The internal structure of the body is designed to compensate for most stresses; however, at times stress becomes too much for the body to handle. Stress can lead to disease if certain functions within the body are inhibited. Massage helps to reduce this interference by inhibiting the depleting effects of stress while promoting proper system function.

Causes of Stress

Stress can come from outside the body in the form of physical stimuli like cold, heat, noise, or the lack of oxygen. The body can generally remain in balance, because it is built to deal with these environmental changes. However, at times these physical stressors create more of a response than the body and mind can deal with. For example, too much heat can cause heat stroke or exhaustion as well as a shift in the emotional response, appearing as impatience, even rage. Stress can also come from your social environment, such as the demands of work or family, creating undue stress on the internal environment. Or stress can begin internally, perhaps as an inflammation or low blood sugar, but eventually the mind and emotions become involved too. Eventually, many stress-related issues can turn into physical complications. Massage can relax the body and mind, help prevent illness, and support good health. In Chapter 8 you learned more about the causes of stress and the body's response. Here you will learn how to use massage for specific stress-related issues.

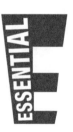

The continued use of massage as a preventive measure for stress works because it calms the mind as well as the body. Massage works to release the built-up tension in the muscles that causes stiffness and lack of mobility. Relief from these symptoms frees the body to relax and move, and releases the mind from thinking about feeling stiff and sore.

Headaches

There are a variety of reasons why you might have a headache. Muscle tension in the neck and shoulders that is left unattended will cause a headache. A sinus infection can bring on a terrific headache. People who clench their jaws are prone to headaches. Migraine headaches and cluster stress headaches can be severe and painful. At times eyestrain may bring on a headache.

Massage can help relieve the pain of headaches and sometimes eliminate the cause of headaches. Become aware of your body and understand the warning signs of certain types of headaches. Pay attention to your neck, shoulders, and upper back. If you feel tension and tightness in the muscles in those regions it is time for a massage. Ideally you should keep your body limber and tension free, so you can stay ahead of the aches and pains. A simple routine to relieve or prevent headaches looks like this:

1. Place your hands on either side of your face, thumbs in and fingers resting on your temples, and circle gently over your entire forehead up into the hairline; repeat.
2. Circle with your fingers along your jawline from your chin to your ears, working along the edge and following up with an easy pinching stroke using your thumbs and index fingers.
3. Circle with your fingers on your cheeks, working around the cheekbones up to the sides of your nose; press with your fingertips along the bridge of your nose.
4. Gently pinch along the ridge of your ears from the lobes up to the tops of your ears and back to the lobes again, stroking down the earlobes with your thumbs and index fingers; repeat.
5. Shampoo your head working your entire head from the back of the skull, along the sides to the top of your head; circle in the ridges at the base of your skull.
6. Circle down the back of your neck, feeling the tight muscles under your fingers; then knead along your shoulders as far as you can comfortably reach and feather off.

The more you practice this simple routine on yourself, the more release of tension you will have in these areas. This will also help relieve sinus headaches, although prevention of sinus-related infection involves managing your diet as well.

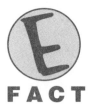

Abdominal Issues

Ulcers, gastritis, irritable bowel, and stomachaches are a few of the digestive disorders that may be the result of emotional distress. Nicotine, caffeine, alcohol, and anti-inflammatory medicines can also trigger the formation of ulcers. Some folks are genetically predisposed to developing these abdominal problems; however, if these folks manage to release tension and work through their stress, they often do not suffer any symptoms. Proper eating habits and regular practice of stress management work to prevent many of these conditions. Not surprisingly, massage is a wonderful antidote as well as a preventive method for dealing with these problems. A full-body massage, a chair massage, or a self-massage are all techniques that support the organs of the abdomen and release stress that may be held in that region.

Problems with the Respiratory System

Respiration begins when you inhale through your nose. The air moves into your lungs where oxygen is passed into the blood and circulated throughout your body. When you exhale, you breathe out the carbon dioxide that your blood has returned to your lungs. This respiration process is continuous.

Polluted air, smoking, exposure to chemicals, and airborne allergens can affect the quality of your breathing. Massage contributes to the health of the respiratory system by supporting the exchange of oxygen and carbon dioxide in the lungs, as well as respiration on a blood and cellular level. Exercise, proper breathing, and a nutritious diet also help maintain the health of your respiratory system.

Often when people experience breathing problems, whether from a cold, allergies, or infection of the nose and sinuses, they find it difficult, if not impossible, to lie facedown while they receive a massage. Ask the recipient if he or she prefers to lie facedown, or with the face turned to the side, or if it is better to turn the entire body to the side as you work on the back. Chair massage is another option for someone with breathing issues. Whatever feels comfortable for the receiver will work. Of course if your massage partner is experiencing painful breathing or shortness of breath, encourage that person to seek medical attention.

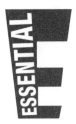

Respiration also takes place at the cellular level where cells pass gaseous waste to the blood in exchange for oxygen and other nutrients. Oxygen is added to the other components in the cell in a process known as oxidation.

Minor Aches and Pains

The relief of aches and pains may have been your introduction to massage, as you searched for a way to feel better when those bones and muscles began to ache. The causes of these pains can cover a wide spectrum, and only a medical practitioner can really assess the causes. But minor aches and pains caused by overuse, misuse, and under use all respond well to massage. Frequent massage encourages the blood flow to the muscles and surrounding nerves, promoting their strength and flexibility, and helping them to thrive.

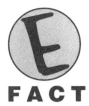

It is important for you to know that you can massage someone with osteoporosis (a degenerative bone condition), although you need to modify your technique by using less pressure and slower, easier movements. Diet, nutritional supplements, weight-bearing exercise, and massage all contribute to the prevention of bone loss.

Massage relieves muscle spasms and tension, relaxing stiff muscles as circulation improves. The soreness you would normally sustain from overused muscles dissipates with frequent massage. Massage also helps with the healing of bone disorders, such as fractures that are in recovery. While the body is healing from the break, massage of the rest of the body is helpful in the whole body process.

Chronic Pain

Chronic pain is debilitating physically, mentally, emotionally, and spiritually. If you suffer from endless pain you know that much of your life revolves around how to deal with it. You wake up in the morning in pain, spend all day dealing with the pain, and go to bed and sleep (if you are lucky), still in pain. Pain is the body's way of letting you know that something is not balanced. Unfortunately many people ignore the pain unless it is a major injury that must be addressed immediately. We are a society that has learned to use the "grin and bear it" option when dealing with our pain. Even worse, for many of us, our pain has been addressed as though it were "all in your head."

Pain is real, whether it stems from an injury, an illness, overuse, or emotions. The pain that you feel is real. Doctors might not know why you are in pain, so you ignore it until it becomes too big for your life, at which point you are in a chronic state of pain. Steady, unrelenting pain will wear you down. No matter how strong you are, your inner reserves will be swallowed up and diminished if you spend them all on chronic pain.

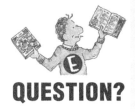

QUESTION?

What is a chronic state?
A chronic state is a condition that continues over a long time period and may bring about a severe change within the body. A chronic condition is always present, creating a debilitated state in the body. Long-term stress is chronic and can result in disease.

There are two classifications of pain: acute and chronic. Acute pain is sharp pain with a sudden onset. It can be caused by anything from a pinprick to a knife cut. Chronic pain, on the other hand, is a slow-acting pain that begins gradually and increases in intensity. The type of feeling associated with this pain is aching, throbbing, and burning. Examples of chronic pain would be the pain of arthritis or an untreated toothache. Unfortunately, some people suffer from conditions such as chronic pain syndrome (CPS) and fibromyalgia, which cause the body to be in pain for no medically known reason (although science is trying to catch up).

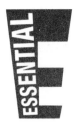

The cause of chronic pain conditions such as CPS is unclear, but whatever the cause, until recently the treatment of choice has been to medicate, using stronger and stronger drugs to either reduce the pain or block the awareness of the pain sensation. Today relaxation techniques, including massage, are helping to lessen chronic pain.

Cardiovascular Problems

Heart disease is more prevalent today than ever before. Issues with the heart are generally compounded by lifestyle, whether the cause is genetic or stress related. Lack of exercise and foods high in bad fats and bad cholesterol weaken the muscles of the heart and overtax the blood vessels. It is now well documented that cardiovascular conditions are best treated using a combination of medical and complementary therapy. Aerobic exercise is an important part of heart disease prevention; working the muscles of the body to elevate the heart rate and increase metabolism helps to keep the heart healthy. This type of exercise brings more oxygen to the muscles and prepares the body to release waste at a quicker rate.

The principals of Swedish massage enforce movements toward the heart, improving circulation and assisting the heart in its work. Massage improves the flow of nutrients through the body by assisting the movement of blood and lymph through the vessels, and helps to eliminate toxins. Each type of stroke has its own important way of helping improve circulation. Effleurage enhances the movement of blood through the vessels close to the skin and in the muscles. Petrissage works with the veins and arteries, stimulating the flow of blood deeper in the body. Friction strokes work to increase the movement of the interstitial fluid as well as the circulation of lymph.

Using Massage for Cancer Patients

Cancer is an extensive subject because every system in the body can develop cancers particular to that system. But the many different diseases associated with cancer have a common denominator: the breakdown and alteration of cells, and subsequent duplication of cancerous changes to other cells. The newly mutated cells invade and erode the healthy surrounding cells, perpetuating the growth of the cancer.

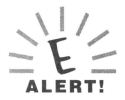
ALERT!

Although most research supports the use of massage on cancer patients, massage that stimulates the circulatory system may assist the spread of cancer. Before administering massage to a person with cancer you must get medical clearance.

If given with the proper medical clearance, massage can be very beneficial to cancer patients. Massage helps deal with the pain related to the disease and lowers the stress level of the recipient. Blood pressure is lowered as the anxiety of the receiver decreases and muscle tension is released. Massage helps to support the natural function of the body to access the disease-killing cells, therefore helping the body to fight cancer.

Massaging Someone with AIDS

AIDS (acquired immune deficiency syndrome) is an infection that stems from a virus known as the human immunodeficiency virus, or HIV. The HIV virus attacks the immune system and destroys the body's ability to fight disease. The HIV virus attacks the infection-fighting T cells on a search-and-destroy mission. As the virus spreads, it systematically seeks out and destroys the T cells, thereby destroying the body's ability to eradicate the virus. Once the immune system is disabled, the HIV virus opens the body to a host of infections, and this condition of heightened susceptibility is the disease known as AIDS.

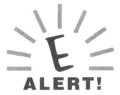

ALERT!

AIDS is spread through the exchange of bodily fluids, period. Not through casual contact or sweat but through semen, breast milk, blood, and vaginal secretions. The person most at risk during a massage is an AIDS-infected receiver, not the giver, because the receiver is so susceptible to infection. The giver must be healthy so as not to compromise the already weakened state of the recipient.

Massage can be administered to someone with HIV at any time, but circulatory massage is not recommended for someone in advanced stages of AIDS. However, other forms of bodywork, such as Reiki, reflexology, and trigger-point therapy can be used for pain and stress reduction. Overall, massage is a wonderful tool for providing compassionate touch, particularly to a population that is still misunderstood. Kind and loving touch will provide comfort and support, and will ease some of the worry and fear related to this disease.

Massage can help with the relief of symptoms of many conditions—if you are not sure, ask your medical practitioner. Most medical advisors recommend some form of massage as a relaxation tool, a stress reliever, and a pain releaser. The important factor in offering massage is your intention. Wanting to give support and care is the key ingredient; you can't go wrong with love in the recipe. Go ahead and give comfort, be it a back rub or a hand massage—you will help bring joy and encouragement to whomever you are massaging.

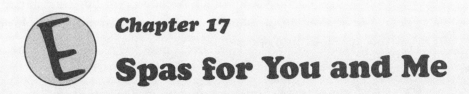

Chapter 17

Spas for You and Me

Massage has come a long way and at the same time still retains many of its historical features. The ancient baths of athletes and royalty, which often included the luxury of a foot soak in sliced lemons and essential oil or an herbal body wrap, are precursors of the modern-day spa. Today spa therapy is being reintroduced as the ideal way to relax and unwind. The richness of a week, an overnight, or at least a day of healing bodywork is available to everyone.

The Evolution of the Spa Experience

Every culture in history has the shared knowledge of the healing properties of water. Natural springs are the focal point of many ancient world communities, supporting the custom of curative baths. Massage and water therapy have been linked from the beginning of history. The Greek and Roman baths, the Native American sweat lodges, the Turkish baths, as well as centers built around healing springs represent the rich history of the use of massage in a spa setting.

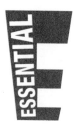

The use of water in healing work has been documented throughout history. The gymnasiums of Greece treated both men and women with water therapy and massage to promote health, heal disease, and ease sore muscles.

Natural springs, which can be either hot or cold, generally contain minerals with healing properties for many physical and emotional conditions. Traditionally spas were built near such natural springs or salt water where the healing properties of the water could be combined with supporting therapies such as massage.

Soldiers Bring Massage to Europe

The connection between water and healing crossed all institutions, from hospitals to the military. French soldiers returning from Turkey introduced the use of massage and healing baths to Napoleon in the 1800s. Soon this concept spread throughout Europe.

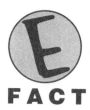

FACT

Napoleon stayed battle-ready with healing baths and massage. The French use of aromatherapy is seen with his choice of oils both in his bath and for his massage. Napoleon would infuse the bathwater with citrus and follow his bath with a lemon-oil massage.

Water therapy and massage were used to help soldiers wounded in battle, either physically or through shock. Spa treatments were provided in hospitals for them and others suffering from different kinds of physical and mental illness.

Sanitariums and Spas

From the 1800s on, the use of water and massage continued to grow in popularity as a means to treat illness throughout Europe and the United States. One important use for sanitariums and spas, though somewhat misguided, was for the treatment of "female feebleness." Nervousness and weakness were considered to be the illnesses of women, curable only with rest and relaxation, so sanitariums and spas were established strictly for this purpose. Often these facilities treated women whose behaviors were not acceptable to society at that time— women who refused to be submissive or who wanted to be educated. Staying at a sanitarium or a spa was often the only way a woman could find respite from the tensions of her normal environment.

Fortunately, not all spas were established as asylums for insubordinate women. Spas began to surface for the benefit of many different classes and types of people, from the affluent to the ordinary folk. Today there are many such resorts and spas that offer water treatments and massage for the health and well-being of anyone looking for relief from physical or emotional stress.

What Spas Offer

The spas of today can be as simple as your own hot tub or as prestigious as the Canyon Ranch Spa in the Berkshires of Massachusetts. Either way, the idea is the same: to promote health and wellness and to treat yourself right, through exercises, nutrition, spa treatments, and massage. You go to a spa to get an organized jump start if you need one, and to experience some healthy pampering at the same time. You might go to a spa for a facial or a seaweed body wrap, or to take a yoga class or enjoy a hot-rock massage. Your spa journey may be in the town you live in, halfway around the world, or right in your own backyard, depending upon what you need and can afford.

Spas come in all shapes and sizes, for all price ranges and tastes, and often have themes that offer experiences in more than simple relaxation. Some types of spas you may want to try are:

Yoga retreats
Family spas
Holistic healing centers
Fasting, juicing, and cleansing spas
Golf spas
Smoking cessation clinics
Weight management centers
Alternative lifestyle spas
Hot springs and mineral baths
Ranch spas

Treatments You Can Choose

Spas offer a wide variety of treatments to pick from. In addition to receiving traditional water therapy and various types of massage, some people like to be wrapped in a special concoction of seaweed and minerals or honey and peppermint or some other exotic mixture. Others enjoy receiving facials with herbal cleansers and tonics that deeply cleanse and refresh the skin. Still others enjoy body scrubs that remove all the dead skin and leave them feeling invigorated.

Nutrition at the Spa

Spas deal with whole health—how your body looks and feels from the inside out. If you go to a spa for a day or more, expect to eat healthy foods that support the concept of proper nutrition. Spa cuisine usually focuses on fresh, low-fat foods and limited meats. Unhealthy fats, sugars, starches, and alcohol are generally no-nos. Some spas focus on seasonal meals or foods native to the region. But all spas focus on foods that support heart health and the immune and digestive systems, and foods that help you detoxify.

You can prepare some of the same foods at home and enjoy healthy spa eating. This is an example of a spa menu:

- **Breakfast:** Yogurt with strawberries and granola; juice or water
- **Morning snack:** Potassium juice (juice together three carrots, two celery stalks, one cup of spinach, one cup of parsley, and one teaspoon of liquid mineral)
- **Lunch:** Lots of salad: romaine, mesclun, radish, sprouts, broccoli, mushrooms, almonds, and brown rice with a dressing of balsamic vinegar and olive oil
- **Afternoon snack**: A fresh fruit smoothie, or a plate of raw vegetables and yogurt dip
- **Dinner:** A protein such as grilled salmon, tofu, or chicken served with two types of lightly steamed vegetables, followed with a ricotta-blueberry sundae and herbal tea
- **Evening Snack:** A cup of cottage cheese, or three slices of turkey, or popcorn

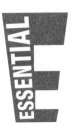

A ricotta-blueberry sundae is simple to prepare. Use ½ cup of part-skim ricotta cheese, and stir in a tablespoon of honey. Then add ½ cup of fresh blueberries or any berries you like. Sprinkle grated coconut and walnuts or almonds on top. Yummy!

The Application of Water: Hydrotherapy

Hydrotherapy is a popular form of treatment. Therapeutic baths are found in salons and spas, and water treatment is used in physical therapy. Immersion in water of the whole body or part of the body provides a valuable healing modality as the water conducts the temperature effectively into the body. You use water therapy yourself anytime you take a soothing, scented bath or a long, warm shower to help release your tension, relax your muscles, and wash away what ails you. Today's spas provide many forms of water therapy and massage to provide relaxation to the entire body and mind.

The Therapeutic Effects of Water

Immersion in hot water raises the temperature of your body and improves your circulation. Because your body is buoyant in water you feel less pressure on your joints and muscles, which helps release pain and tension. Most hydrotherapy tubs have a whirlpool or jet spray component that sends out a stream of water to surround and massage your body. Water massage also stimulates the production of feel-good neurotransmitters (endorphins), allowing for total relaxation.

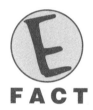

FACT

Endorphins are the body's natural painkillers. They are chemical messengers in the brain that have druglike, pain-suppressant qualities. One way these chemicals are accessed is through stimulation of the skin, which is why massage can help relieve pain.

Therapeutic baths can help provide relief from chronic conditions such as insomnia or nervous tension. In addition, the water encourages the release of toxins as well as additional benefits to the circulatory and elimination systems.

Body Shampoo

Cleansing baths using friction help rid the skin of dead cells. Washing the skin with a brush or mitt, such as a natural loofah sponge, encourages the dead surface cells to loosen and leave the body. The friction application promotes the growth of new skin and provides a vigorous stimulating effect on the skin. By using aromatherapy soap along with friction, you add the soothing benefit of the herb or oil used in the preparation of the soap.

The Effects of Cool Water

Cool baths reduce pain and swelling because the coolness desensitizes the nerves and causes surface blood vessels to contract, pulling the blood away from the swollen area. The body responds quickly to the effects of cold water, so cool baths are generally short in duration. However, the benefits of cool water bathing continue after the bath, providing warmth and increased function as the blood vessels expand again, causing improved circulation. Overused and taut muscles respond to the use of cold water therapy.

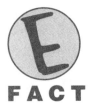

FACT

Cold application in the form of cold wet towels or covered ice packs helps muscle spasms and muscle fatigue. Initially the application of cold reduces the sensitivity of the nerve response, acting like a form of anesthesia. With the removal of the cold water the nerve sensitivity returns to normal, helping restore homeostasis in the body function. Cold application helps muscle spasms and muscle fatigue. Overused and taut muscles respond to the use of cold water therapy.

Whirlpool or Friction Baths

Two other kinds of baths found in spa treatment are the whirlpool bath and the friction bath. Whirlpools are found everywhere—even your local hotel may have a mini-whirlpool next to the regular heated pool. The whirling of the water helps your circulation as well as aching muscles. The gentle agitating pulse of the water on your body is soothing to your nervous system.

Some spas offer what is known as a friction bath. This is a bath given by hand by an attendant. The attendant applies cold water with a wet towel or loofah mitt and briskly rubs part of the body, say the arm, with the water-soaked mitt; then, using friction again, dries the arm with a towel before moving on to the next part. This is a stimulating and energizing bath that you can even do on yourself.

Create Your Own Spa

Think about what you would like to have in your own private spa. Your bathroom can be converted anytime you wish to an exotic mineral spring or plush day spa. Regardless of where you are, you can create a healing space to work your own brand of spa magic.

Transforming a Bathroom into a Spa

To create your own special space, begin with a complete cleansing of your bathroom until every corner, nook, and cranny is washed, dusted, and polished. Change your shower curtain and bath mat to give your bathroom a fresh, new look. Pick soft, light colors. Clear out any clutter, getting rid of old soap ends and partially empty bottles of shampoo. Put everything under the sink or in clear plastic containers that look pretty and stack easily. Take out those pretty towels you have been saving; this is the time you have been saving for. Gather three baskets of various sizes: one for your pretty towels, one for your brushes and loofah mitts, and one for your essential oils and herbal blends. If you don't already have baskets somewhere at home, you can often find them at area yard sales.

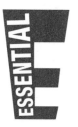

Dry face towels make good friction items and facial brushes. If you do wish to purchase a loofah mitt or sponge, they are inexpensive and can be found at your neighborhood pharmacy or health food store. Essential oils can be purchased at these stores as well.

Selecting Candles, Creams, and Essential Oils

Scented candles enhance the spa atmosphere. Choose colors and scents that appeal to you; often the colors replicate the smells. Pick scented creams that complement and support the aromas you are choosing. If you like lavender-scented purple candles try using a peppermint cream to further support the soothing qualities of the lavender.

When choosing your essential oils or scented creams and candles, take time to think about the qualities you are looking for. If you are interested in oils with a calming effect then you might be interested in chamomile, lavender, lemongrass, rose, or neroli. Oils that stimulate the mind are peppermint, rosemary, mandarin, and clary sage. Oils to make you feel refreshed are chamomile, bergamot, orange, jasmine, and sandalwood. Notice how some oils, such as chamomile, are interchangeable. Essential oils have many different properties and qualities that allow the oils to be effective in many ways.

Homemade Treatments for Your Home Spa

Now that you have created a home spa, you will decide what treatments you would like to experience. You may try a long soak in the tub, or an invigorating shower. Maybe you will give yourself a facial. How about a dry friction rub? You have a variety of techniques to consider. You may use one or, better still, try them all.

Something you might want to try is creating your own spa treatment products. You already know which fragrances and essential oils please you so you can easily take the next step toward being creative. You might even decide to share your new spa and give one of your treatments to someone you love.

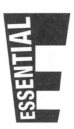

Essential oils work best when added to a carrier oil, such as jojoba, sunflower, or soy oil. The carrier helps to dilute the potency of the essential oil and allows you to minimize your expense. Essential oils also make great skin toners when you blend the aromatic oil with distilled water or vinegar.

Homemade Oatmeal Facial Cleanser

An easy, old-fashioned remedy for face cleansing is made from oatmeal and honey. Long-cooking oats work better than instant oats, but whatever you have in the pantry will do. Use one cup of oatmeal and combine it with one or two tablespoons of honey, and either one-eighth cup of almond oil or eight drops of orange oil (these are essential oils, not the kind from the baking section in your grocery), or another stimulating essential oil. If you have dry skin, try using both the orange oil and the almond oil. Add five or six drops of distilled water or witch hazel and stir until all the ingredients are mixed. This face cleanser will remove the dirt and excess oil from your skin while leaving your natural facial oil. Use it once a week for a deep cleansing.

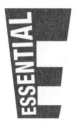

A facial toner is used after you wash your face. You can make your own toner with essential oil of peppermint or lavender. Use up to twenty drops in a small bottle of witch hazel or distilled water. Essential oil of orange works well too.

Creative Facial Masks

Facial masks are often used after deep cleansing to tighten and tone the skin. While daily use of a toner is recommended, masks are used less often. A simple recipe for a mask is an egg white. One egg white applied over your face and left on for fifteen minutes will tighten up your skin and leave you with a smooth feel. Another old remedy mixes a tablespoon of honey into a whipped egg white. This variation should also be left on for fifteen minutes, then rinse off with cold water. Add strained fruit and essential oil to your egg-white concoction, and you create a more sophisticated facial mask that will exfoliate the skin, helping to prevent wrinkles. Essential oils such as orange, neroli, and bergamot are good choices to combine with fruit, and will provide an enhancing addition to your facial mask.

Make Your Own Creams and Oils

A facial and body cream is also easy to make. A few folk remedies combined with aromatherapy give a new twist to an old healing art. Everyone wants a peaches-and-cream complexion and this recipe really helps.

Cook up a batch of soft, too ripe peaches and mash them through a strainer. Sir together one-half to one cup of the strained juice and one-quarter cup less of dairy cream. Add six to twelve tablespoons of brewed chamomile tea along with a few drops of witch hazel. Stir until smooth and pastelike in consistency, then apply. This cream will soak right into your skin helping to relieve any dryness you may feel. Make enough to use on your whole body, and refrigerate any leftovers.

Scented oil for your body and your bath can be made with essential jojoba or almond oil as the carrier. Have a small plastic bottle cleaned and ready. Fill a small bottle with the carrier oil and add six drops of chamomile oil, plus four drops of neroli or bergamot oil. Shake well before massaging your arms, legs, and torso with the oil. Use six drops of the blended oil in your bath or add only the essential oil to your shower gel.

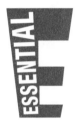

The complimentary bottles containing shampoo and cream rinse that you receive when you stay in a hotel make perfect bottles for your oil, and you will be recycling as well. Or pick up some inexpensive plastic travel bottles at the drugstore.

Spa Shopping

You have designed your own spa and prepared and used your own products, so now you have a clearer picture of what you would like in a spa. Basically the way to pick your spa is to decide how long you want to be involved with the experience, what exactly you want to receive, and whether or not you want to travel.

Day Spas

Perhaps the closest and most accessible to begin with is the day spa. Day spas usually offer therapies similar to those offered by "stay" spas. You can get anything ranging from water therapy to aromatic massage— but you will not be staying overnight. These are great places to receive a fantastic massage, get your face and hair done, get a manicure or pedicure, and more. Some day spas even provide classes and holistic health care. Some provide chiropractors, childcare, bridal services, maternity massage, and other holistic offerings. Day spas are providing one-stop shopping for preventive health care.

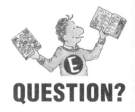

With so many spa choices how do I decide?
The spa experience you choose will depend on what you are looking for. Decide if you want to lose weight, meditate and eat macrobiotic foods, actually bathe in a mineral spring, or just be pampered. Then, call around to see who offers the specific things that will help you relax.

Stay Spas

Some stay spas are part of a larger resort, while others exist as their own separate retreat. Either way these are places where you might stay one night or as long as a week or more. Some stay spas offer other experiences, such as sports activities, as part of the package. These spas are called "experience spas" and are becoming more popular all over the world as more choices are being offered. The stay spas that deal with only spa treatments may offer a day of cleansing hydrotherapy and massage, followed by an herbal wrap and a reflexology session. Every day would build on the detoxification and release of the previous day.

Whether you choose to enjoy yourself in the comfort of your own spa or treat yourself to a dedicated spa experience, you will feel cleansed in body, mind, and soul. Take a moment to contemplate and breathe, spritz the air with an infusion of orange blossom, take a long hot bath with a few drops of lavender, live for a time in the spa. Close your eyes and feel the warmth permeate every cell in your body, savor the quiet, and become one with the energy of the experience. Ⓔ

Chapter 18

Specialized Massage and Body-work Techniques

The different forms of massage and bodywork—the techniques and the benefits unique to each one—are rooted in the cultures that developed them. The techniques we use today come from those developed in China, Japan, Thailand, India, and Sweden, to name just a few. Whenever you give a massage you use a combination of techniques that are connected to a variety of bodywork systems, many of them ancient.

The Foundations of Eastern Medicine

Traditional Eastern medicine principles are based on the concept of the uninterrupted flow of life force through hundreds of meridians and acupressure points in the body. The idea that yin and yang energy exists within the body is also an essential component of this belief system, which teaches that the opposite poles of yin and yang must be in alignment for the body to function at its highest capacity. Understanding the principles of the life force, meridians, and yin and yang is an important first step in understanding the actual massage practices that grew from them. The application of these principles is found in the assessment and treatment of the whole body, physical and energetic.

The Life Force

The life force, or vital force, is the energy that is present in you and all around you. Everything consists of energy; only the packaging is different. Think of it as something similar to The Force that Luke Skywalker learns about from his master Yoda in the *Star Wars* movie series. The harmonious flow of this life force maintains a natural level of all body functions, including emotions and spirit. The disorder of energy can disrupt health and the feeling of well-being.

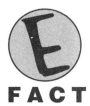

FACT

Ch'i or qi is the Chinese name for your vital life force, the energy of the universe that flows through you and all matter, and the thread that connects us all. In Japanese culture it is known as ki, in India it is prana, and in Tibet it is lung-gom.

Meridians

Energy flows through the body along an uninterrupted path of interconnected channels called meridians. The meridians are the pathways through which the vital life force flows. Traditional Chinese medicine makes use of these channels through acupressure and acupuncture to balance the energy flow within the body, stimulating the healer within and allowing the body to heal itself.

There are twelve pairs of main meridians and eight meridians known as vessels. The meridians run on either side of the body, six beginning or ending in the hands and six beginning or ending in the feet. The meridians are connected to organ functions as well as the elements of nature and the balance of yin and yang. The vessels form a conduction system that provides fuel for the channels and feeds the body at large. The twelve main meridians are located as follows:

Lung	Bladder
Large intestine	Kidney
Stomach	Gall bladder
Spleen-pancreas	Pericardium
Heart	Liver
Small intestine	Triple burner

The energetic functions of the main meridians are the same as the functions of the organs they connect with; treat the points along a meridian and you treat the organs related to the energy line. Other meridians are related to multiple organs, such as the triple burner meridian that runs through the center of the body and is responsible for heating the organs. In massage, acupressure applied by the fingers works specific points on meridian lines, either concentrating on one point or moving through the entire meridian line, depending on the massage.

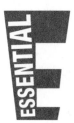

Meridians circulate ch'i just as blood flows through arteries and veins, lymph flows through lymph vessels, and nerves follow a pathway. All of these circuits travel continuously throughout the entire body through every system, from one organ to another, through every body part, promoting balance.

Yin and Yang

Yin and yang are central concepts in traditional Chinese and Japanese medicine. The qualities of yin and yang are complementary and mutually dependent; they represent the duality of nature. Yin represents the female force, and yang represents the male force. Yin is the feminine passive principle in nature that in Chinese cosmology is exhibited in darkness, cold, or wetness; yang is the masculine active principle in nature that is exhibited in light, heat, or dryness. Together, yin and yang combine to produce all that comes to be. Because you are part of the universe, you have these opposing, yet balancing, forces within you. In the body, the internal regions are yin and the external regions are yang. For example, the muscles and bones are yin and the skin is yang. Looking from a physiological standpoint, yin stores the energy and yang performs the activities. The goal of Eastern treatment is to balance yin and yang by opening the flow of energy along the channels and restoring harmony.

The Five Elements

According to Chinese thinking, five elements make up the world: metal, water, wood, fire, and earth. These are the natural forces essential for life. Although termed "elements," these categories deal with the energy forces that are the conditions of being. You are comprised of these five elements, because you are part of nature. Imagine a wheel, a continuum of energy that has no beginning and no end. The elements are such entities that one element flows along the circle producing another element and so on. The relationship between these elements within your body represents the quality of your health.

Traditional Chinese Medicine

The system of traditional Chinese medicine (TCM) consists of four methods of treatment: herbology, manual therapy, acupuncture, and food treatments. Through thousands of years of study and application, the principles of this system have been used to maintain good health and prevent disharmony. TCM focuses on the cause of the discomfort or illness rather than the symptoms. Chronic pain and illness respond dramatically to this form of healing. The classic Chinese medical book, *The Yellow Emperor's Classics of Internal Medicine* (University of California Press, 2002), or *Nei-Jing,* was originally published in the third century B.C. and documents the whole spectrum of Chinese medical arts. Today traditional Chinese medicine and modern Western techniques are used together in China, and the value of this integration is starting to be accepted in the West as well.

Acupressure

Acupressure is applied pressure through finger and thumb movements to specific points on the energy meridians. This ancient Chinese method of healing is the model for many other pressure-point therapies, such as shiatsu and tui-na. Pressing the meridian points on the receiver's body, from the fingertips to the feet and along the lines between the meridians, sends messages to the brain along the meridians. A fully clothed receiver lies on a mat as the giver presses the points along the energy meridians. This gentle, noninvasive work relieves stress, relaxes the body and the mind, improves blood circulation, relieves muscle aches and pains, aids in the removal of toxins, and encourages whole body health. Acupressure deals with the receiver as a whole being—every point connects to every other point within the body, and all these points connect to the mind and spirit as well. Acupressure works to restore homeostasis; as the body is balanced, harmony returns.

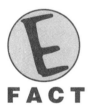

FACT

Moxibustion is the application of heat on specific acupuncture points. The moxa is a long thin stick of rolled herbs that when lit sends the healing properties of the herb into the body. Cupping uses heated glass cups placed along meridian lines to draw toxic waste from the body to the skin surface, where it can be washed away.

Tui-Na

The bodywork system of tui-na uses a variety of techniques from traditional Chinese medicine, including massage, joint mobilization, acupressure, moxibustion, and cupping. This system uses a combination of these techniques in a variety of ways, depending upon the need of the receiver. The flow of energy, ch'i, is considered and the meridians are used to restore balance. Tui-na is often used in conjunction with foods and exercise to promote true healing. A tui-na practitioner diagnoses the recipient by feeling his or her pulse. Today doctors in China study tui-na along with acupuncture and herbs.

A recipient of tui-na is fully clothed except for his or her shoes and lies on a mat. Of course the recipient relates any painful conditions before the work begins. The giver works on acupressure points, the meridian lines, and the muscles and joints of the receiver. Tui-na relieves sore muscles and joints, produces a feeling of calm, and at the same time renews energy.

The Japanese System

The Japanese system of healing is based on many of the concepts found in the traditional Oriental medical philosophy. The Japanese method of healing uses the basic Oriental precepts of yin-yang, the five elements, and meridians. The balance of ki, the life-force energy, is elemental to the work of shiatsu, the Japanese system of finger pressure. In shiatsu, pressure is applied to tsubo points located along the meridians. The response of the nervous system is a total body/mind reaction. Traditional Japanese medicine also involves Kampo treatment, the medical use of herbs indigenous to Japan.

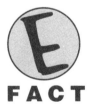
FACT

Tsubo is the exact point on a meridian where shiatsu is applied. When pressure is applied to the tsubo point, underlying congestion is dissipated and harmony is restored through improvement the flow of ki, the vital force. Proper application of pressure brings internal and external balance.

Shiatsu

Shiatsu is the Japanese word for finger pressure. Shiatsu uses finger and hand pressure, combined with gentle manual manipulation of the body, to work with the life force, ki, to promote healing. Using the principles of Oriental medicine, shiatsu works toward whole health, and its goal is to bring the opposite poles (yin and yang) into balance while restoring the flow of ki. The process involves the pressing of tsubo points along the meridians, which are the energy lines that access every organ and body part. This form of touch appears simple in action, but requires great skill to enlist the vital life force to come into balance. Every point that receives pressure calls out for harmony throughout the body, mind, and spirit. Regular sessions of shiatsu teach the body to recognize harmony as the desired state of being.

Fully clothed, the receiver sits and then lies on a mat or cushion while the giver presses points along the energy lines. The giver also stretches and rotates certain areas of the receiver's body as part of the routine. The release of toxins, tension, and energy blocks leaves the receiver of shiatsu feeling relaxed and energized when the session is over.

Kampo

The Kampo system of herbalism, which has been time-tested over more than a thousand years, uses particular herbs to treat specific symptoms. The particular herbs deal with the individual's response to the illness (the symptoms), not the cause or cure of the illness itself. Kampo deals with a person's sho, which is the person's response to emotional, physical, mental, spiritual, and social conditions. To bring a person's ki back into harmony, his or her sho must be in balance.

Herbs are administered in combination or singly, depending upon the state of the client's sho. There are hundreds of formulas to match every condition of sho that may surface. Generally, Kampo formulas have no serious side effects, making a Kampo treatment seem more desirable than many drugs. The herbs used in this system have many active ingredients, allowing for better use of the primary ingredient while leaving very little chance of toxic reaction. Some Kampo practitioners provide a shiatsu treatment along with herbal treatment; others will refer the receiver to a qualified shiatsu practitioner.

Thai Massage

Traditional massage from Thailand has its roots in history dating back 2,500 years. The "Father Doctor" Jivaka Kumar Bhaccha, an Indian devotee of Buddha, is credited with the development of Thai massage. In early times, Thai massage was used to treat many different aliments such as liver and respiratory disorders and muscle weakness. Today, Thai massage is used to treat soft-tissue and muscle soreness, to restore mobility in these areas, to reduce stress, and to restore balance. Recipients of this massage feel renewed and strong with increased energy.

Today, this massage is beneficial in treating soft-tissue and muscle soreness as well as helping to restore mobility. Thai massage helps to reduce stress and restore balance. The recipient is fully clothed for a Thai massage session, sans socks. Thai massage is provided to the receiver on a mat. The giver uses a stretch to open the session. The giver then uses thumbs and palms to press certain points along the energy lines of the body. The application of sustained pressure on specific points along the meridian lines opens up the energy channels. The practitioner continues from the points to a series of stretches that support the release of blockages and keep the energy flowing. Recipients of this massage feel renewed and strong with increased energy.

Ayurvedic Tradition

"Ayurveda" is translated as "the science of life," to know how to live in health, The ayurvedic tradition for perfect health includes the concepts of meditation, yoga, massage, nutrition, and herbal medicine. The principles of ayurvedic wisdom come from 5,000 years of work and study in this ancient Indian tradition. The process involves body-mind education and healing by influencing the nervous system. Its purpose is to reunite the individual self with the higher self, or pure conscious self.

Balancing prana, the universal life force, brings inner harmony and well-being. Ayurvedic treatment works on the pranic level first, then moves into the physical. As the energy of the prana is worked, the nervous system begins the healing process, sending a message to the physical, which sends a corrected message to the brain.

Ayurvedic thinking supports positive wellness, with no room for negative thoughts, feelings, or behaviors. The freedom to be whole and healthy is within all of us, and it is up to each of us to take the steps to find freedom from pain, disease, discomfort, and fear. We all have the ability within us to be free from all limitations. All is possible. The practices of yoga, meditation, and guided visualization are essential to ayurvedic thought. The use of herbs externally and internally is also an essential part of the ayurvedic tradition, as is eating simple yet elegant foods, which feed the body as well as the soul.

Yoga

Yoga is the ageless system of healing that is integral to the ayurveda thought. Yoga teaches us to be centered and to focus on the moment. Yoga teaches us how to breathe correctly, and how to use our breath to get the most from our bodies. In a sense, yoga uses our breath and bodies to train our minds and bodies to perfect health.

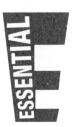

Yoga is a way of life. Once you begin to consciously and responsibly practice yoga, your life will change for the better. As you breathe properly and understand the movement of your body, you begin to embrace the divine within. You recognize through facing your own weakness that we are truly all the same.

Ayurvedic Massage

The concept of ayurvedic medicine comes through in the ayurvedic system of massage. Ayurveda means the science of life and its purpose is to provide a lifestyle that will provide whole health through understanding how the mind influences the body. This principle promotes self-awareness of body and mind. Balance is the recipe.

Balance of body, mind, and spirit is promoted through the basic concepts of right diet, thought, exercise, intention, giving, and compassion. Massage is an important part of the health care with this system. A self-massage before you bathe in the morning is recommended to help rid the body of toxins and stimulate the system.

Ayurvedic massage is a tool to use every day, with oil or without. Massage your head as though you were giving yourself a shampoo, and then use long gliding strokes down your body, over your chest, as much of your back as you can reach, and finally your arms and legs. Rub your feet between your hands and press on your toes. This is a wonderful way to begin your day, and even better if you do some yoga stretches before the massage. The balance of energy and structure are essential for you to be the whole and powerful being that you are. Bodywork and massage help to keep us in balance, and restore us when we tip.

Other Ancient Traditions

The art of healing touch has been passed down from generation to generation by a variety of different cultures. Several of these traditions remain today, proving just how beneficial these massage techniques can be.

Reflexology

Reflexology is an ancient form of healing touch that is physical and energetic and that classically exemplifies the greater world of bodywork. More than a foot rub, not a massage, this work uses thumbs and fingers to apply pressure to specific points on the feet, hands, and ears that represent the greater body. By working these points, zones, and meridians on the feet you will affect the whole body. When you work on the sole, you touch the soul.

Each foot has more than 7,000 nerve pathways that flow through the body to the brain and then from the brain to other parts of the body. Through the use of reflexology the giver can release stress, promote circulation, and help remove toxins. At the same time, the receiver relaxes on such a deep level that when the treatment is finished, the receiver feels trouble free. Reflexology continues to work long after the touch has ended, helping to keep the receiver stress free.

Reiki

Reiki is energy healing work. Dr. Mikao Usui, a Buddhist monk and spiritual teacher who studied and traveled the world searching for a powerful healing tool, reintroduced this ancient form of touch. This healing work is applied following a systematic pattern that connects with the chakras. After a program of study, the practitioner may either place her hands directly on the receiver or lift her hands up into the aura.

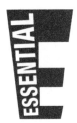

Your aura is the field of energy and light that surrounds your body. Research from the University of California reveals the existence of rays of color emanating from the fingertips of people. Changes in emotions reflected changes in color as observed in the photographs from the study.

Reiki calms the nerves, reduces stress, and promotes overall relaxation. It helps to diminish pain, and restores energy and vitality to the receiver. Reiki is so simple that a child can practice this loving form of healing, yet Reiki is so powerful it can seem miraculous. Documented cases show Reiki combined with conventional medicine can relieve many symptoms and assist in the healing process. Reiki connects you with your divine energy, allowing you to give unconditionally, with kindness and compassion.

Lomilomi

Lomilomi is a traditional form of Hawaiian healthcare, originally known only by the indigenous families of Hawaii. It is a native form of medical massage used to work on injuries and muscle tension to relieve muscle spasms, increase flexibility, improve circulation and respiration, stimulate the central nervous system, and help with digestion. The concept of this healing technique is to touch upon the ability of the receiver to heal him- or herself. Medical practitioners may refer a client to a Lomilomi practitioner. This integrative and complementary treatment is recognized as helpful in the treatment and recovery of illness and injury and, as such, is often covered by health-care insurance.

The Swedish Method of Massage

This method is the mainframe of modern-day massage. The Swedish system of massage takes into account anatomy, physiology, and the way the body's functions and systems respond to particular manipulations and strokes. Swedish massage utilizes the movements that come naturally to humans—glides, kneads, pinches, twists, presses, taps, pulls, shakes, and stretches—to work on the soft tissue and underlying muscles, releasing toxic waste and promoting circulation. Swedish massage is the number-one choice for stress reduction. Athletes want this form of massage because it stimulates their muscles before an event and releases the knots and tension after an event.

Swedish massage can be soft and gentle, deep and firm, and stimulating, all at one session. This type of massage is very effective for chronic pain, because the strokes can be used to reach deep into the tissue, releasing adhesions while teaching the muscles new memories of how to function properly. The main physiological effects of Swedish massage are the relaxation and stimulation it provides to the muscles, the circulatory system, and the endocrine system.

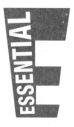

The strokes of Swedish massage increase circulation, help reduce swelling, and help release toxins from the body while at the same time relieving tightness and pain from the muscles. A greater sense of well-being is promoted through this release. If you feel better physically, you feel better mentally and emotionally.

Swedish massage improves skin tone because improved circulation of the blood increases the oxygen supply that feeds the skin. The nervous system benefits also, whether slowing down or speeding up, depending upon the individual need of the body being massaged. Swedish massage is beneficial in almost all instances, although some conditions do need to be cleared through a medical practitioner.

Deep-Tissue Massage

Deep-tissue massage is the application of a variety of strokes that affect the deep tissues and fascia of the body. This massage is directed toward the supportive and protective layers of fascia—the layers covering the entire muscular system—to keep these layers moving freely. Deep-tissue massage techniques work to release the physical tension and restrictions in the muscle tissue, encouraging mobility and freedom from pain. These physiological procedures are often combined with psychological release brought about by the deep bodywork as the pressure opens old restrictions. The work of deep-tissue massage actually changes the physical structure of the body, aligning the core of the body both physically and emotionally. The idea is to realign the structure of the body by improving posture and releasing restrictions in the muscles. The spine and muscles hold the memories of proper body function as well as past trauma, so to fix the spine and the structures that support it means fixing the whole body.

The Trager technique is a form of deep structural integration developed by Dr. Milton Trager. The Trager technique teaches the receiver to relax as mobility is regained. There are two parts to this method. The first is a series of rhythmic stretching and rocking movements administered by the giver, who shakes the parts of the receiver's body that are constricted, such as tight muscles and painful joints. The point of this movement is to produce a state of deep relaxation. Secondly, the receiver learns a number of movements to practice at home. These movements support the relaxation and mobility that the giver has introduced.

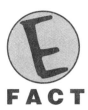

FACT

Dr. Trager developed his famous technique long before he became an M.D. As a young gymnast and dancer Trager would receive massage from his coach. The young Trager began to experiment with his own style of massage, first on his amazed coach and then on his father. The technique that Trager developed freed his father of severe sciatica in two sessions.

Rolfing is a form of deep-tissue massage named for its developer, Dr. Ida Rolf. Rolfing helps to align the spine and body so that the organs will function properly. Dr. Rolf discovered that poor posture from childhood creates a misalignment that causes long-term problems such as poor body structure, poor muscle tone, and interference with the functions of the internal organs. Rolfing reshapes the body's posture as well as realigning the muscles and connective tissue. This deep work is performed with fingers, knuckles, closed fist, or an elbow.

The role of massage and its many variations continues to grow in acceptance. As you learn about and start to practice various techniques, see if you can feel the differences. Some are subtle and some are obvious. Let your hands and fingers continue to guide you on this limitless journey of touch. E

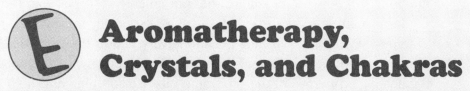

Chapter 19

Aromatherapy, Crystals, and Chakras

The sense of smell and the sense of touch are essential to the work of massage. Every day we breathe about 23,000 times, inhaling and exhaling a multitude of scents contained in the air. Some scents are part of daily life; others are introduced for therapeutic purposes. Certain fragrances can reduce blood pressure and help you to deal with stress and panic. Other scents can speed up your metabolism, keeping you at peak performance. The aromas that you choose to use on your body can provide many wondrous experiences.

The Uses and Benefits of Aromatherapy

Aromatherapy uses medicinal-quality essential oils derived from plants. These oils offer assistance in restoring energy and strengthening the immune system. Although oils for aromatherapy are most commonly associated with the sense of smell, they can also be applied directly to the body. The tiny oil molecules that are quickly absorbed into the tissues of the nose are also absorbed by the skin, especially through the feet. Within twenty minutes from application every cell in the body will be infused with the essence, and the nutrients will begin working, spreading the healing properties of the oil. Some oils are soothing and help to reduce anxiety. Others stimulate the body and provide an energy boost. Essential oils affect the hypothalamus and pituitary gland, influencing the endocrine system and the production of hormones.

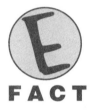

FACT

Essential oils are antioxidants. Antioxidants interrupt the damage that can be caused by free radicals, fungus, and cell mutation. Aromatic essential oils are antibacterial, antiviral, and antiseptic, and they work against infection and destroy parasites. These oils can also destroy odors while removing toxins from the air.

Essential oils are used not only to calm the mind and emotions, but also to support body functions. Essential oils can fight and at times destroy bacteria and even viruses. Oils work to restore homeostasis. The chemical properties of essential oils have vital components that work against many of the disease-causing organisms. The use of oils provides support to all the body systems, and they can make you smell good, too.

The Origins of Aromatherapy

The ancients used scents derived from plants for medicinal and cosmetic purposes, and history of their use is found in all cultures. Written documents in China speak of the medicinal properties of over 100 varieties of plants. Artifacts from ancient China show the use of incense for worship ceremonies and in honor of the dead. Traditional Ayurvedic medicine from India uses aromatic plants for medicinal purposes as well as food. Hindu mythology has many references to aroma, and essential oils were used for incense as well as for embalming. The traditional use of incense and essential oils was practiced in Japan as well. Incense is still used in all these cultures.

The Influence of Egypt

Egypt is credited with further developing the use of essential oils, moving from not only religious ceremonies and embalming but also the use of oils in cosmetics. In the year 2800 B.C. a school for the study of plants was founded, and people from that school later established laboratories in the temples to prepare the sacred oils, incense, and perfumes. A great trade business for oils was established between Egypt and other regions; the raw materials were imported to Egypt, and Egyptian tradesmen refined the oils, later returning the finished product in trade.

Egyptian perfumers developed new processes to produce essential perfumes. One method involved steeping flowers or oils in animal fat, giving the fat the scent of the oil. This product was molded into cones and used to perfume wigs. Another process called for chopping the elements, then cooking and straining them, storing the resulting oil in alabaster jars to be used for creams and perfumes. A third method required pressing the flowers to extract the oil, which was used for perfume. Dry powders, known as unguents, were also produced and kept in jars to preserve their aroma. Some of these jars still contain fragrance twenty-two centuries later.

Middle Eastern Developments

The Middle East was a source of many of the plants used for producing essential oil, and the process of extracting oils from the plants through distillation was developed there. The use of essential oils was studied extensively in Arabia, which shared its findings on using oils for incense, cooking, and medicine with the rest of the world. Ancient records in Babylon show the use of oils in medical treatments as well as religious ceremonies. History reports that the Queen of Sheba traveled with gifts of oils and spices as gifts for King Solomon of Jerusalem.

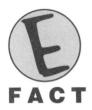

FACT

The ancients of North and South America used fragrance in their medical practice and religious ceremonies. Aromatic plants from these regions were used to treat illness as well as to provide comfort. The essential oils from the plants were also used in the ceremonial practices, through incense and perfumes.

Aromatic Oils in the Bible

The Bible has many references to the use of fragrant oils in the Old Testament. Oils were used by the Hebrews in almost all of their sacred ceremonies. The book of Exodus tells of Moses learning to make incense and holy oil, and each book of Moses (the first five books of the Old Testament) carries lessons in the preparation and use of fragrant oils. The early kings of Israel, including King David, were anointed with oil. In the New Testament, the Wise Men present the newborn Jesus with gifts of essential oil, and throughout the New Testament are many further references dealing with the use of oil for anointing.

Greek and Roman Contributions

No discussion of ancient culture is complete without reviewing the impact of the Greek and Roman empires. The Greeks studied plants for their medicinal qualities as well as for the aromatic perfumes they could produce. The famed Greek physician Hippocrates, the father of medicine, recognized oils as medicinal and recommended daily aromatic massage. The Greek physician Galen used oils in his practice and study of medicine. Romans continued the use of oils derived from plants, producing many physicians and scientists who studied plants and their usage.

How to Use Essential Oils

The application of oils is simple. The most common way is with a diffuser. Diffusers allow particles of oil to be scattered through the air and inhaled. With the use of essential oils, less is more. Two or three drops in a bowl of hot water or a cold water spray is usually enough to disperse the scent throughout a large room. The aromatic and healing properties of the oil will work for hours. Bathing is another way to feel the effects of the different oils and wear your favorite scent all day long. Remember to always dilute your oils.

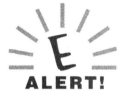

ALERT!

Essential oils are medicinal and you must follow certain guidelines. Do not use oils undiluted, and do not use them on anyone with cancer, a high temperature, a skin infection, or a childhood disease. If you are pregnant, consult a professional aromatherapist. Use only natural oils, not synthetic ones.

Using Oil for Massage

Oils are used in massage after they have been diluted with a pure carrier oil—jojoba oil is a good choice. The quickest way to feel the effects of essential oils is through the feet. The reflexology points in the ears are also a good place to apply oil. To decide which oil you like best, give it a sniff test. Open the bottle, let the oil sit, and allow the fragrance to permeate the air. Close your eyes and inhale; see if you experience anything. While inhaling the scent, make sure you . . .

- Like the smell.
- Do not feel sick.
- Can breathe comfortably.
- Feel good all over.
- Do not get a headache.

Also make sure that no one else in the room experiences any negative effects from the oil, especially your massage partner. Once you have had a successful test of the oil you have picked, you can begin.

An Easy Foot Massage

Massaging the feet is a fun and easy way to experiment with the use of aromatics, because feet are one of the best diffusers of oil, spreading the healing properties through the entire body. Let your receiver rest comfortably face up in a lounge chair, on a blanket, or on a table. Carefully place bolsters or pillows under the receiver's knees and behind the head if needed. Cover the receiver with a light blanket because temperature of the body drops when we relax. Take off the receiver's socks and wash the feet.

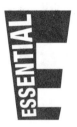

The olfactory cells in the nose are replaced every thirty days. Tiny hairs called cilia respond to the different odors in the air and stimulate these cells. Olfactory cells trigger old memories because they connect directly with the section of the brain that relates to feelings, wants, and creativity.

Rub some oil between your hands to warm it up, and apply some to the right foot first with smooth strong strokes. Then apply some to the left foot with the same strokes, and cover the left foot with a towel. Back on the right foot, glide from the toes to the ankle and from the heel to the toes, using both hands at the same time if you wish. If working top and bottom together is too awkward, just work on the top of the foot first and then the bottom.

For this next movement, use your thumbs first on the top of the foot and then on the bottom of the foot. Walk from side to side across the top of the foot using your thumb, covering the entire surface while your fingers hold the bottom of the foot. Switch hands and walk your thumbs across the sole of the foot, covering the entire surface. Now squeeze and press with one of your palms along the sole of the foot and up one side. Switch hands and work on the other side of the same foot.

Next, make your hand into a fist and press gently into the sole of the foot from the heel to the neck of the toes and back again. Grasp the foot with both hands and gently shake, letting the energy run up the leg. Release the foot and, using both hands, gently feather off the top of the foot with your fingertips. Cover the right foot with the towel and work the whole routine on the left foot. When you have completed both feet cover them and rest your hands on top of them.

Crystals and Chakras

The body has many layers: physical, intellectual, emotional, and spiritual. You feel things physically but also on an emotional and spiritual level, too. In the Hindu teachings, this interaction of layers is explained with the idea of chakras. The Sanskrit word *chakra* means wheel. Each wheel is an energetic center that spins in our bodies, dealing with some aspect of our health and well-being. Although there are hundreds of these energy wheels spinning within us, the best known and most significant are the eight chakras that run parallel to the spine.

The chakras spin all the time and each one is associated with color, emotions, and specific physical functions. In fact, each chakra is associated with a particular gland in the endocrine system. These wheels are the transmitters of energy, and they disperse the collective energy of the universe into your body for you to use

What Are Crystals?

Crystals are elements of the earth that have been used for centuries in healing. Crystals are gemstones that are made into jewelry, used in oils, or simply placed in a window to reflect light. The colors of the stones are assigned to different chakra wheels and, as such, are used together in specific pairings. Many people wear crystals and gemstones because they are pretty and they reflect the color that the person is working with at the time. The color is reflected from the chakra and whatever issues are apparent.

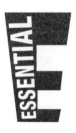

Universal energy is the concept that we all are connected through the shared energetic current that vibrates through the universe. This energy is composed of different layers—spiritual, emotional, intellectual, and physical. The force outside our body is referred to as the divine energy.

The Root Chakra

The root chakra is the base of the chakras and is found at the tailbone. The color of this chakra is red, and it is connected to the adrenal glands and the fight-or-flight response. The root chakra's function is to keep you grounded: to keep your feet firmly planted on the earth, focused on survival. The physical ailments connected with this chakra are constipation, fatigue, joint and bone problems, and stress-related conditions. The crystals connected with the chakra root are ruby, onyx, hematite, red jasper, garnet, smoky quartz, and black tourmaline.

The Sacral Chakra

The sacral chakra is the second chakra and it is found at the sacrum. Its color is orange and it is linked with the ovaries and testes, dealing with sexuality and sensuality as well as reproduction. The physical conditions connected with the sacral chakra are muscle spasms, allergies, sexual imbalance, infertility, and lack of creativity. The crystals and stones are amber, citrine, topaz, moonstone, and fire opal.

The Solar Plexus Chakra

The third chakra is the solar plexus chakra, which is found in the center of your abdomen just above your belly button. Its color is yellow and it is connected with the pancreas and adrenal glands. Here you deal with self—this is the seat of the soul, and it is the place from which you form your opinions. Physical imbalance with this chakra results in exhaustion, gallstones, diabetes, digestive problems, ulcers, and allergies. The crystals here are peridot, yellow topaz, watermelon tourmaline, yellow tourmaline, citrine, amber, and tiger's eye.

The Heart Chakra

The heart chakra is found at the heart, and its color is green. This chakra deals with emotion, love, compassion, kindness, balance, and giving. The problems caused by imbalance here could be respiratory issues, heart attack, high blood pressure, insomnia, depression, fatigue, anger, tension, and general negativity. The stones connected with this chakra are emerald, jade, malachite, aventurine, and diopside.

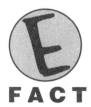

FACT

Aura-Soma is a form of therapy developed in the 1980s that uses color, essential oil, and minerals to create a healing tool that combines the essence of light with the stability of the earth. This therapy involves bottles of brightly colored oil, each containing specific healing properties.

The High Heart Chakra

The high heart chakra is located between your heart and your throat and it is directly over the thymus gland. Its color is pink and it is connected with the energy of the divine. Here you find your spiritual base, that part of you that wishes to meditate, pray, and help others. This chakra deals with your faith. The problems connected with this chakra could be insufficient production of T cells, HIV, and early onset of aging. The crystals connected with this chakra are rose quartz, coral crystal, and watermelon tourmaline.

The Throat Chakra

The throat chakra, located in the throat, is connected with the thyroid and parathyroid glands. Its color is blue, and this chakra is about expression, communication, responsibility, and speaking universal truth. Problems connected with this chakra are speech impediments, respiratory problems, headaches, pains in the neck and shoulders, throat problems, difficulty communicating, ear infections, and lack of creativity. The stones for this chakra are aquamarine, turquoise, sapphire, blue quartz, and lapis lazuli.

The Third Eye

The chakra known as the third eye is found between your brows and is linked with the pineal and pituitary glands. The third eye deals with your inspiration, spirituality, awareness, and intuition. The color is indigo. Problems with this chakra can be eye and ear diseases, nose and sinus problems, headaches, and nightmares. The stones for this chakra are sugilite, fluorite, amethyst, and azurite.

The Crown Chakra

The crown chakra is found on the top of your head, at the crown. The colors connected to this chakra are purple, gold, and white. Here is your direct connection to your higher self, to the divine, to your guardian angels. This is the center that looks at your spiritual beliefs: how you think and feel about that reality. Physically this chakra is connected with the nervous system and the pituitary gland, and perhaps all of the endocrine system. Headaches and depression are connected with this chakra. The crystals that go with the crown chakra are amethyst, diamond, and clear quartz.

Hot Rock Massage

Hot rock massage works with the chakra system, utilizing stones. The stones are heated in warm water to bring soothing heat to the area of each chakra and the surrounding areas. Generally the stones are river stones or basalt stones, or you can use any stone you find on the beach or the riverbank. Try to find smooth, flat ones starting about three inches in diameter on down to about one inch around. You'll need about ten to fifteen altogether. Some people prefer to use crystals that reflect the color of the chakras. Whatever you choose, the basic concept is to stimulate the area through the use of the stone. An added benefit is that the stone does the work, not your hands. To prepare the stones, place them in a glass container with hot water and leave them to soak, allowing the heat to penetrate into the stones.

With your receiver lying facedown, place a large flat stone, about three inches in diameter, on the root chakra, at the base of the spine. Follow up the spine, gently placing a warm stone at each chakra, picking smaller stones as you move up the body. Once you have positioned the chakra stones you can use a warm round stone that fits into the palm of your hand to gently glide up the calves, stopping just below the knee. Glide up over the calf muscle on both legs and then move to the buttocks.

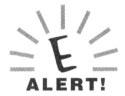

Always use a slotted spoon or prongs to remove the stones. Do not reach your hand into the hot water, and be sure to check the stones before placing them on the body of your recipient. If you cannot comfortably hold the stone do not put it on your receiver. When the stone can be held comfortably it is ready to be used.

Gently glide over the hip and glute region, exchanging stones when the one you are using becomes cool. Feel how easy and smooth the movements are and make sure to check with your receiver about your pressure; do not press too hard. Remove the stones from the chakra areas and use a warm stone in your palm to glide over the back muscles. Do not glide directly on the spine or neck. To complete the session use your fingertips to gently stroke over the back, and then press your hands firmly on the shoulders to indicate that this massage is over. Hot rock massage tones and stimulates, relaxing the muscles while the heat penetrates deeply into the muscle bellies.

Aromatic essential oils, crystals, energy wheels, and color combine to give you a wonderful experience. The world of massage is as wide as you wish it to be, with many exciting avenues waiting to be explored. Follow what interests you and there will be more to explore on this infinite journey. Ⓔ

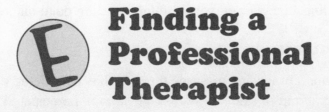

Chapter 20

Finding a Professional Therapist

Receiving is as good as giving. You have been busy giving everyone you know a massage, and now it is your turn. Now that you have tasted the richness of giving, it is time to feel the joy of receiving. Once you know where to look, you will find many different places to receive a massage, and many types of people who give them. Along the way you may find that you want to become a massage therapist yourself; if so, congratulations!

All Therapists Are Not Created Equal

You need to keep several things in mind when searching for your ideal therapist. You want to be sure the therapist is qualified and knows what he or she is doing. It is also important that you like the way that particular therapist works. The glowing recommendation of a friend is not enough—you may find that your personal preferences are quite different.

Checking Credentials

At the minimum, a practicing massage therapist has completed a 400- to 500-hour program of study at a massage school, participated in a clinical internship or study, passed a written and practical exam, and maybe also worked as an apprentice before striking out on her or his own. After a massage therapist receives certification from a massage school, stating that the recipient is proficient in the professional field of massage therapy, the therapist applies for a license to practice in the state where he or she lives. Once the therapist completes the required exams for licensing, the therapist is qualified as a certified professional practitioner of massage.

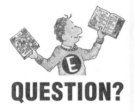

QUESTION?

What credentials are there beyond certification and a license?
Membership in professional organizations indicates the therapist is dedicated and serious enough to be a member of a governing group that upholds certain standards and ethics. Also, additional postgraduate study indicates that this therapist loves the work and is continuously refining his or her skills.

When you begin your search for the right massage therapist, refer to the checklist and find out how many hours of training the therapist completed, if there was a practical requirement, if the therapist is certified by the school he or she attended, and if the therapist is licensed. If your town requires licensure this should be posted along with the certification from the practitioner's school.

Personal Taste

It could be that the best massage you've ever had came from a man who works in your gym and received his training from his aunt, who received her training from her grandma, and so on. It may not be a wall full of certificates that ultimately convinces you that someone is the best massage therapist for you. Let your personal preference be your guide. Go with what feels best for you, physically, emotionally, and spiritually.

Equally important is the therapist's philosophy of massage therapy and bodywork. A therapist's philosophy is the set of beliefs, values, and standards that guide his or her work. The ethics of massage are straightforward and true: to treat everyone with compassion, honesty, and respect, and to uphold the professional guidelines of healing at all times. Talk to a potential therapist to get a sense of whether he or she upholds these values.

Choosing the Type of Treatment

What is the right treatment for you? The answer to this question may change every day, because you do different activities every day and the needs of your body can change. To assess what the best treatment is for you, begin with what you like. If your preference is for deep muscle massage, consider how your body feels today as you move and exercise. How do your neck, shoulders, and back feel? Are your muscles tight or fluid? Tight areas in the large muscle groups respond well to a deeper massage, but the muscles of your neck may need something different. The right treatment for you is what feels good and what helps you to improve your feeling of well-being. Stay open to new things and rely on your therapist to help you decide on the best treatment.

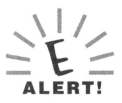

ALERT!

When you answer your massage therapist's questions, be up front with your answers, especially when it comes to medical issues. Your massage practitioner will base your session on what he or she observes and on what you say. It is important to reveal honestly the state of your health and how you feel overall.

Where Are You Coming From?

A trained massage therapist will help you determine what is the best treatment for you. Discuss with the therapist how a day in your life typically runs, exploring your energy level, your physical strengths and shortcomings, as well as what you expect to gain from your treatment. Together you will decide if relaxation is the primary goal, or relief from chronic pain, or a combination of these, calling for a variety of treatment styles.

What Are You Looking For?

If releasing stress is a primary goal, the massage therapist will address your tense muscles as well as your inability to relax. As the therapist begins to massage, you will feel anxiety and depression begin to fade away. The more relaxed you become the deeper the strokes will go, soothing you to the core. Deep massage work is not necessarily painful, because as the body releases tension, it opens up to change on a deep level without resistance. A good massage therapist understands this.

If you want more flexibility in your muscles and joints, again the massage professional is qualified to work through a series of strokes and massage styles that will best provide what you want. As the restricted tissues are released, the therapist may work deeper or lighter depending upon what your body is saying. Deeper work often releases buried emotions as well. Whatever your needs, the sense of contentment and deep release from massage will leave you glowing.

Looking for the Right Place

You know what you are looking for in a therapist and you know what you need, so where do you look for a therapist? Massage therapy is offered in beauty salons, department stores, at your gym, or maybe even at your office. Many therapists work at the offices of medical practitioners, such as chiropractors, acupuncturists, and naturopaths. Where to go to get a massage is an individual decision; do some exploring to find which of these environments is right for you.

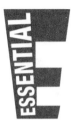

Some massage practitioners prefer to bring the table to you. If that's what you choose, then your job will be to create a comfortable workspace for the therapist, so you receive your massage in a peaceful and serene setting. Let others in your household know that massage time is your sacred time.

Massage and the Beauty Business

Many beauty salons recognize that taking care of yourself through massage is just as much a form of support as taking good care of your hair and nails. You stay healthier and feel better when you look good, and salons provide that service. Many beauty salons now offer spa treatments as the business of wellness becomes more inclusive. It is possible that the place where you get your hair and nails done has a massage service, too, so check it out.

Massage as an Allied Health Profession

Many medical practitioners offer massage in their office. Your chiropractor knows that you will stay adjusted longer and receive the work easier if you have regular massages. Other medical practitioners may prescribe massage as a form of relaxation and for pain relief. Still others recognize massage as a complement to whatever treatment they are providing.

Massage Clinics

Massage schools hold clinics for their students to practice on all types of bodies. Clinics cost less and provide a broad spectrum of choices for you, the consumer. With such a variety to choose from you can experience many different touches and techniques. Contact your local massage school to find out when the school holds its clinic.

Massage in the Mainstream

With the growing acceptance of massage, don't be surprised if you find an opportunity for therapy in the middle of your daily routine. For example, maybe your favorite perfume counter sponsors a five-minute chair-massage demonstration right in front of the counter to promote the latest scent. Or perhaps you come across a permanent chair-massage booth at the airport where, for a dollar a minute, the therapist massages you while you wait for your plane. Stress is everywhere and massage is here to help de-stress people on their way through life.

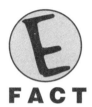

FACT

Many massage schools also sponsor days of wellness where you can attend and receive whatever services are offered on that day. Generally a day of wellness is a community service program and operates by donation.

What to Expect

You found where you want to have your massage and made an appointment with the therapist you like. Today is your first appointment and you are wondering what will happen. Besides the fact that you are going to have a great massage, some other pieces of business need attention.

Your massage therapist will greet you and then ask you a series of questions. These questions will range from information about your name and phone number to your medical history, allergies, and whether or not you are taking medication. You may also be asked whether there are certain areas of your body that are painful and what your expectations are— what benefits do you expect to receive from the massage? These questions are important for helping the practitioner understand how to proceed, and if any extra precautions need to be taken. Always answer honestly.

Training in Massage Therapy

Out of the hundreds of hours of training a therapist receives, generally 50 percent of it is hands-on, while the other half is spent receiving massage. The philosophy is: To give a good massage, a therapist must know what a good massage feels like. Today the requirements also include a profound understanding of how the body and mind work in harmony.

A massage professional is trained to be a life coach, a keen observer, and an excellent listener. Massage therapists are trained to know when to refer clients to a medical professional, and how their work complements other therapies clients may be receiving. The commitment of massage professionals is to support the wellness model within their own lives as well as those of their clients.

As you know by now, massage therapy is more than rubbing backs. And it is more than getting paid for helping people feel good. Massage therapy is a complement to every part of life, from birth to death and all that is between. Massage is holistic—working hands-on you help heal mind and body by providing relaxation and relief from stress, pain relief, better circulation, and detoxification. Massage therapists are highly trained professionals who love their jobs and relish the comfort and relief they provide to others. The commitment to perform massage is a way of life.

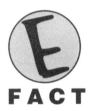

FACT

Massage training throughout the world requires the student to complete high school (or its equivalent) before moving on to massage school. A student must have basic skills in order to handle the requirements of advanced training in massage, its techniques, and the physiological responses of the body.

The Course of Study

The study to become a professional practitioner of massage includes courses in anatomy and physiology as they relate to massage, in pathology, and in health and safety. There is a course in business that generally covers making a business plan and preparing for entry into the world of professionalism. Universal precautions for the health and safety of the practitioner and the client are part of every massage program. Preparing therapists also study the ethics of behavior, which deals with how to interact professionally while adhering to a strict code of values and conduct. In addition, aspiring massage therapists learn clinical documentation as it pertains to the profession, and how to make professional assessments that allow them to provide the best service for their clients. Students of massage also study its history.

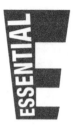

Following school certification a postgraduate goal is to achieve the national standard by successfully completing the national massage exam, offered by the National Certification Board for Therapeutic Massage & Bodywork.

The profession of massage recognizes the growth in its industry and sets standards and qualifications, which are recognized in this examination process.

Studies in massage continue after graduation, with the therapist choosing to expand his or her knowledge and mastering techniques in other bodywork methods.

The field of massage and bodywork is expanding and becoming increasingly more accepted as a field of complementary medicine. Massage allows us to touch with compassion and give the receiver a feeling of love and safety. Massage allows people to take some quality time for themselves, away from the hustle and bustle of everyday life. Whether you are giving or receiving, make time to enjoy the healing benefits of the wonderful art of massage. (E)

Appendix A: Glossary

abdomen: The structure in the center of the body that holds the visceral organs; the center of the life-force energy, or ch'i.

acupressure: A form of traditional Chinese medicine in which fingers are used to press into the energy points on the meridians to promote healing by releasing congestion and allowing the life force, or ch'i, to flow clearly.

acupuncture: A traditional Chinese medicine practice that uses needles inserted into energy points along the meridians to promote wellness; the points are energetically connected to the organs of the body and the needles free congestion to bring balance and harmony.

adrenal glands: The hormone-producing glands that sit on top of the kidneys.

adrenaline: The main fight-or-flight hormone produced by the adrenal gland.

anatomy: The study of the structure of the body.

anatripsis: The art of rubbing the skin up toward the heart using the flow of the circulatory system to rid the body of waste; discovered by Hippocrates.

anma: The original form of massage healing used in ancient China.

aromatherapy: A therapeutic treatment using medicinal-quality essential oils.

Avicenna: The late tenth-century Persian doctor who authored *The Canon of Medicine,* a book that classifies, describes, and presents the causes of innumerable diseases.

ayurveda: An ancient Indian form of medicine that combines yoga, meditation, massage, and herbal medicine to promote a healing lifestyle.

baths: Used today to promote healing and relaxation with water; originated in ancient times.

bodywork: Any form of touch that uses techniques to bring about change and healing; not necessarily massage.

chair massage: A seated massage with the person fully dressed; can be performed anywhere and can be as short as ten minutes.

chakras: Energy points within the body that keep a sense of balance through connections with the endocrine and central nervous systems.

ch'i: A term used in Chinese healing that represents the vital life-force energy in the body.

chiropractor: A doctor of natural medicine who treats the spine to heal the body.

connective tissue: Tissue that supports and binds together other tissues, and includes such fibrous tissue as tendons, ligaments, and cartilage; it provides support and protection while holding everything in the body together.

connective tissue massage: Deep massage that helps rid the body of toxins in the muscles, joints, and organs.

deep-tissue massage: Swedish massage as it is used to work deep into the fascia to free restrictions in muscle tissue.

drape: A form of covering used during massage to allow the receiver to feel safe and secure.

effleurage: A Swedish massage term used to describe long, gliding strokes; this stroke is often the mainstay of the massage.

endocrine system: The system that produces all the hormones of the body.

energy work: A type of bodywork that works with the vital life-force of the body (ch'i) to release congestion and promote balance.

essential oils: Natural oils derived from plants and distilled with steam to reach the essence of the plant; they can be used for medicinal, therapeutic, or cosmetic purposes.

fascia: The fibrous tissue covering the entire muscular system.

fight-or-flight response: Our instinctual response to an emergency that tells us to fight off the enemy or flee; produces increased blood pressure, heart and respiratory rates, and skeletal muscle blood flow, all of which is not useful in most present-day stressful situations.

friction: A massage stroke that moves the skin over the muscle, releasing tension and breaking up adhesions.

Galen: An ancient Greek physician and a prolific writer who used massage in his work.

gymnasium: An institution of ancient Greece where athletics, massage, and debate took place; the model today is the spa.

hammam: The baths in Arabic countries.

Hippocrates: Considered to be the Greek father of medicine, he has influenced medicine throughout history; Hippocrates was the first to use anatripsis, a type of rubbing.

homeostasis: The state of equilibrium; the preferred state of the body.

hydrotherapy: Any water therapy; a direct descendant from the Greek gymnasium.

interstitial fluid: The fluid in between the cells and blood vessels.

ischemia: A condition where the blood flow to the muscles is constricted, causing pain.

ki: The Japanese word for the vital life-force energy.

kneading: A form of Swedish massage, also known as petrissage, that is performed as though you are kneading dough.

ligament: A tough fibrous band of connective tissue that connects bone to bone or keeps an organ in place.

lymph: Fluid that helps feed the cells and is key in fighting infection by taking toxins away from the body.

lymph drainage: A process that helps the lymph system to function, reducing swelling and releasing toxins.

massage: The manual manipulation of the soft tissues of the body.

meridians: The life-force energy channels that run through the body; there are twelve main meridians and six vessels used in acupuncture, acupressure, and many other forms of bodywork.

metabolism: The internal process within your body that transforms food to energy.

muscle fatigue: The condition of a muscle when it has worked so hard it does not respond when contracted.

muscle spasm: The involuntary contraction of a muscle or a number of muscles; can result from the buildup of lactic acid during exercise.

nervous system: The system comprising the brain and spinal cord, nerves, and ganglia that receives and interprets stimuli and transmits impulses throughout the body tissue.

pain: The sensation your body creates to let you know if something is wrong with the function of your body; your body's alarm system.

palpation: The examination of the body by feeling with your hands and fingers, such as in massage.

petrissage: The kneading technique used in massage.

physiology: The study of the functions of the body.

polarity therapy: Therapy that uses massage, energy work, and visualization to balance the body.

prana: The Hindu word for the vital life-force energy.

pressure points: Specific points that run along the meridians and are connected to particular organs; used in forms of therapy such as acupuncture and acupressure.

qi: Alternate spelling of ch'i; the Chinese word for the vital life-force energy.

reflexology: A system of bodywork using points in the feet, hands, and ears to treat the entire body; brings deep relaxation and physical relief from illness.

Reiki: A system of energy work in which the giver works with the receiver's energy field, known as the aura; provides a deep sense of well-being and promotes healing.

Rhazes: An eighth-century Islamic Persian doctor who promoted massage, exercise, diet, and water therapy.

shiatsu: An ancient traditional Japanese finger-pressure treatment; adapted from the Chinese anma and tui-na techniques.

spa: Today's name for a treatment center that provides water treatments, massage, and even healthy food; the modern-day equivalent to the Greek gymnasium.

sports massage: A special massage for athletes using mostly Swedish techniques; given before an event to stimulate, after the event for relaxation, and during training to maintain muscle fitness.

stress: The stimulus that makes the body respond with the production of adrenaline; if the stimulus is not dispelled, the body continuously reacts with a fight-or-flight response.

Swedish massage: The mainframe of modern-day massage; a system of massage that uses movements known as effleurage, petrissage, and tapotement to work on the soft tissue and underlying muscles, which help release toxic waste and promote circulation.

tapotement: The tapping, percussion strokes in Swedish massage.

tendon: Dense fibrous connective tissue that unites a muscle with a bone.

Thai massage: An ancient form of healing that balances the ch'i, using pressure on the healing points and passive stretching.

tui-na: A variety of techniques from traditional Chinese medicine, including massage, joint mobilization, acupressure, moxibustion, and cupping. Evolved from Chinese anma.

tsubo: The Japanese name for the deep pressure points along the meridians.

wellness: The concept of prevention of disease, as opposed to treating the symptom; the wellness philosophy encourages you to take charge of your own continued health.

yoga: An ancient healing system using breathing, diet, and stretching postures to promote wellness.

Appendix B: Resources

Organizations

The following is a list of organizations that can help you find a massage therapist, a good massage school, or massage materials:

American Massage Therapy Association (AMTA)
✉ 820 Davis Street, Suite 100
  Evanston, IL 60201-4444
✆ 847-864-0123
🖉 www.amtamassage.org

American Organization for Bodywork Therapies of Asia (AOBTA)
✉ Laurel Oak Corporate Center
  Suite 408, 1010 Haddonfield-Berlin Road
  Voorhees, NJ 08043
✆ 856-782-1616
🖉 www.aobta.org

American Reflexology Certification Board (ARCB)
✉ P.O. Box 740879
  Arvada, CO 80006-0879
✆ 303-933-6921
🖉 www.arcb.net

Associated Bodywork & Massage Professionals (ABMP)
✉ 28677 Buffalo Park Road
  Evergreen, CO 80439-7347
✆ 1-800-458-2267
🖉 www.abmp.com

Australian Acupuncture and Chinese Medicine Association Ltd.
✉ P.O. Box 5142, West End
  QLD, 4101
  Australia
✆ 07 3846 5866
E-mail: *aacma@acupuncture.org.au*

Dhanvantari Academy
✉ 10 Summer Street, #1109
  Malden, MA 02149
Nimai Nitai Das, Director
✆ 617-413-7259
E-mail: *positiveayurveda@comcast.net*

The Institute for Complementary Medicine (ICM)
✉ P.O. Box 194
  London SE16 7QZ
  England
✆ 00 44 17 237-5165
🖉 www.icmedicine.co.uk

International Council of Reflexologists
✉ P.O. Box 78060, Westcliffe Postal Outlet
  Hamilton, ON L9C 7N5
  Canada
✆ 905-387-8449
🖉 www.icr-reflexology.org

International Massage Association (IMA)
✉ 3000 Connecticut Avenue, N.W. #308
  Washington, DC 20008
✆ 202-387-6555
🖉 www.internationalmassage.com

International Spa Association (ISPA)
✉ 546 East Main Street
Lexington, KY 40508
✆ 1-888-651-4772
✐ *www.globalspaguide.com*

National Certification Board for Therapeutic Massage & Bodywork
✉ 8201 Greensboro Drive, Suite 300
McLean, VA 22102-3810
✆ 703-610-9015
✐ *www.ncbtmb.com*

Books

Here are a few resources on the subjects covered in this book:

Ackerman, Diane. *A Natural History of The Senses.*

Adamson, Eve. *The Everything® Stress Management Book.*

Barnett, Libby, and Maggie Chambers. *Reiki Energy Medicine.*

Beck, Mark F. *Milady's Theory and Practice of Therapeutic Massage.*

Blate, Michael. *The Natural Healer's Acupressure Handbook.*

Borysenko, Joan. *7 Paths to God.*

Brennan, Barbara Ann. *Hands of Light.*

Cailliet, Rene. *Soft Tissue Pain and Disability.*

Calvert, Robert Noah. *The History of Massage.*

Chopra, Deepak. *Perfect Health.*

Clark, Rosemary. *The Everything® Meditation Book.*

Coulter, David. *Anatomy of Hatha Yoga.*

Davis, Phyllis R. *The Power of Touch.*

Devereux, Charla, and Bernie Hephrun. *The Perfume Kit.*

Dougans, Inge. *The Complete Illustrated Guide to Reflexology.*

Eddy, Mary Baker. *Science and Health.*

Franzen, Suzanne. *Shiatsu for Health and Well-Being.*

Fritz, Sandy. *Mosby's Fundamentals of Therapeutic Massage.*

Gach, Michael R., and Carolyn Marco. *Acu-Yoga.*

Goodman, Saul. *The Book of Shiatsu.*

Hamlyn. *Head Massage.*

Heath, Alan, and Nicki Bainbridge. *Baby Massage.*

Inkeles, Gordon. *The New Massage.*

Jackson, Richard. *Holistic Massage.*

Jaffe, Marjorie. *The Muscle Memory Method.*

Jarmey, Chris, and John Tindall. *Acupressure for Common Ailments.*

Judith, Anodea, Ph.D. *Wheels of Life.*

Kirsta, Alix. *The Book of Stress Survival.*

Kushi, Michio, and Edward Esko. *Basic Shiatsu.*

Lidell, Lucy. *The Sensual Body.*

Lidell, Lucy. *The Book of Massage.*

Loewendahl, Evelyn. *The Power of Positive Stretching.*

Loving, Jean E. *Massage Therapy.*

Lu, Henry C. *Chinese Natural Cures.*

Lundberg, Paul. *The Book of Shiatsu.*

Lunny, Vivian, M.D. *Aromatherapy.*

Maxwell-Hudson, Clare. *Aromatherapy Massage.*

McCarty, Patrick. *A Beginner's Guide to Shiatsu.*

McClure, Vimala Schneider. *Infant Massage.*

Mitchell, Karyn. *Reiki: A Torch in Daylight.*

Montagu, Ashley. *Touching, the Human Significance of Skin.*

Mumford, Susan. *The Complete Guide to Massage.*

Muramoto, Naboru. *Healing Ourselves.*

Myss, Caroline. *Anatomy of the Spirit.*

O'Keefe, Adele. *The Official Guide to Body Massage.*

Pritchard, Sarah. *Chinese Massage Manual.*

Prudden, Bonnie. *Pain Erasure.*

Rister, Robert. *Japanese Herbal Medicine.*

Roizen, Michael F. *Real Age.*

Rush, Anne Kent. *Romantic Massage.*

Rynerson, Kay. *The Thai Massage Workbook.*

Salvo, Susan G. *Massage Therapy, Principles and Practice.*

Sharamon, Shalila, and Bodo J. Baginski. *The Chakra Handbook.*

Stillerman, Elaine. *Mother Massage.*

Stormer, Chris. *Reflexology, the Definitive Guide.*

Tappan, Frances. *Healing Massage Techniques.*

Tortora, Gerard. *Introduction to the Human Body.*

Tucker, Louise. *An Introductory Guide to Reflexology.*

Walters, Lynne. *Kind Touch Massage.*

Werner, Ruth, and Ben E. Benjamin. *A Massage Therapist's Guide to Pathology.*

Wescott, Patsy. *Overcoming Stress.*

Yogananda, Paramahansa. *Autobiography of a Yogi.*

Magazines

There are very few magazines dedicated to massage. Here are three:

Massage Magazine
✉ 1636 West First Avenue, Suite 100
  Spokane, WA 99204
☎ 1-800-533-4263

Massage Therapy Magazine
✉ 820 Davis Street, Suite 100
  Evanston, IL 60201-4444
☎ 847-864-0123

Massage Australia
✉ P.O. Box 13
  Windang, New South Wales 2528
  Australia

Web Sources

The Internet is another good resource for information about massage. Here are a few Web sites for obtaining equipment, but there are many more:

✍ *www.allyouknead.com*

✍ *www.isokineticsinc.com*

✍ *www.365fitness.com*

✍ *www.massageoutpost.com*

✍ *www.bestmassagetable.com*

✍ *www.promedproducts.com*

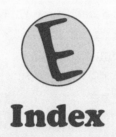

Index

THE EVERYTHING SERIES!

BUSINESS

Everything® **Business Planning Book**
Everything® **Coaching and Mentoring Book**
Everything® **Fundraising Book**
Everything® **Home-Based Business Book**
Everything® **Leadership Book**
Everything® **Managing People Book**
Everything® **Network Marketing Book**
Everything® **Online Business Book**
Everything® **Project Management Book**
Everything® **Selling Book**
Everything® **Start Your Own Business Book**
Everything® **Time Management Book**

COMPUTERS

Everything® **Build Your Own Home Page Book**
Everything® **Computer Book**

COOKBOOKS

Everything® **Barbecue Cookbook**
Everything® **Bartender's Book, $9.95**
Everything® **Chinese Cookbook**
Everything® **Chocolate Cookbook**
Everything® **Cookbook**
Everything® **Dessert Cookbook**
Everything® **Diabetes Cookbook**
Everything® **Indian Cookbook**
Everything® **Low-Carb Cookbook**
Everything® **Low-Fat High-Flavor Cookbook**
Everything® **Low-Salt Cookbook**
Everything® **Mediterranean Cookbook**

Everything® **Mexican Cookbook**
Everything® **One-Pot Cookbook**
Everything® **Pasta Book**
Everything® **Quick Meals Cookbook**
Everything® **Slow Cooker Cookbook**
Everything® **Soup Cookbook**
Everything® **Thai Cookbook**
Everything® **Vegetarian Cookbook**
Everything® **Wine Book**

HEALTH

Everything® **Alzheimer's Book**
Everything® **Anti-Aging Book**
Everything® **Diabetes Book**
Everything® **Dieting Book**
Everything® **Herbal Remedies Book**
Everything® **Hypnosis Book**
Everything® **Massage Book**
Everything® **Menopause Book**
Everything® **Nutrition Book**
Everything® **Reflexology Book**
Everything® **Reiki Book**
Everything® **Stress Management Book**
Everything® **Vitamins, Minerals, and Nutritional Supplements Book**

HISTORY

Everything® **American Government Book**
Everything® **American History Book**
Everything® **Civil War Book**
Everything® **Irish History & Heritage Book**
Everything® **Mafia Book**
Everything® **Middle East Book**
Everything® **World War II Book**

HOBBIES & GAMES

Everything® **Bridge Book**
Everything® **Candlemaking Book**
Everything® **Casino Gambling Book**
Everything® **Chess Basics Book**
Everything® **Collectibles Book**
Everything® **Crossword and Puzzle Book**
Everything® **Digital Photography Book**
Everything® **Easy Crosswords Book**
Everything® **Family Tree Book**
Everything® **Games Book**
Everything® **Knitting Book**
Everything® **Magic Book**
Everything® **Motorcycle Book**
Everything® **Online Genealogy Book**
Everything® **Photography Book**
Everything® **Pool & Billiards Book**
Everything® **Quilting Book**
Everything® **Scrapbooking Book**
Everything® **Sewing Book**
Everything® **Soapmaking Book**

HOME IMPROVEMENT

Everything® **Feng Shui Book**
Everything® **Feng Shui Decluttering Book, $9.95 ($15.95 CAN)**
Everything® **Fix-It Book**
Everything® **Gardening Book**
Everything® **Homebuilding Book**
Everything® **Home Decorating Book**
Everything® **Landscaping Book**
Everything® **Lawn Care Book**
Everything® **Organize Your Home Book**

All Everything® books are priced at $12.95 or $14.95, unless otherwise stated. Prices subject to change without notice.
Canadian prices range from $11.95–$31.95, and are subject to change without notice.

EVERYTHING® KIDS' BOOKS

All titles are $6.95

Everything® **Kids' Baseball Book, 3rd Ed.** ($10.95 CAN)
Everything® **Kids' Bible Trivia Book** ($10.95 CAN)
Everything® **Kids' Bugs Book** ($10.95 CAN)
Everything® **Kids' Christmas Puzzle & Activity Book** ($10.95 CAN)
Everything® **Kids' Cookbook** ($10.95 CAN)
Everything® **Kids' Halloween Puzzle & Activity Book** ($10.95 CAN)
Everything® **Kids' Joke Book** ($10.95 CAN)
Everything® **Kids' Math Puzzles Book** ($10.95 CAN)
Everything® **Kids' Mazes Book** ($10.95 CAN)
Everything® **Kids' Money Book** ($11.95 CAN)
Everything® **Kids' Monsters Book** ($10.95 CAN)
Everything® **Kids' Nature Book** ($11.95 CAN)
Everything® **Kids' Puzzle Book** ($10.95 CAN)
Everything® **Kids' Riddles & Brain Teasers Book** ($10.95 CAN)
Everything® **Kids' Science Experiments Book** ($10.95 CAN)
Everything® **Kids' Soccer Book** ($10.95 CAN)
Everything® **Kids' Travel Activity Book** ($10.95 CAN)

KIDS' STORY BOOKS

Everything® **Bedtime Story Book**
Everything® **Bible Stories Book**
Everything® **Fairy Tales Book**
Everything® **Mother Goose Book**

LANGUAGE

Everything® **Inglés Book**
Everything® **Learning French Book**
Everything® **Learning German Book**
Everything® **Learning Italian Book**
Everything® **Learning Latin Book**
Everything® **Learning Spanish Book**
Everything® **Sign Language Book**
Everything® **Spanish Phrase Book**, $9.95 ($15.95 CAN)

MUSIC

Everything® **Drums Book (with CD)**, $19.95 ($31.95 CAN)
Everything® **Guitar Book**
Everything® **Playing Piano and Keyboards Book**
Everything® **Rock & Blues Guitar Book (with CD)**, $19.95 ($31.95 CAN)
Everything® **Songwriting Book**

NEW AGE

Everything® **Astrology Book**
Everything® **Divining the Future Book**
Everything® **Dreams Book**
Everything® **Ghost Book**
Everything® **Love Signs Book**, $9.95 ($15.95 CAN)
Everything® **Meditation Book**
Everything® **Numerology Book**
Everything® **Palmistry Book**
Everything® **Psychic Book**
Everything® **Spells & Charms Book**
Everything® **Tarot Book**
Everything® **Wicca and Witchcraft Book**

PARENTING

Everything® **Baby Names Book**
Everything® **Baby Shower Book**
Everything® **Baby's First Food Book**
Everything® **Baby's First Year Book**
Everything® **Breastfeeding Book**
Everything® **Father-to-Be Book**
Everything® **Get Ready for Baby Book**
Everything® **Getting Pregnant Book**
Everything® **Homeschooling Book**
Everything® **Parent's Guide to Children with Autism**
Everything® **Parent's Guide to Positive Discipline**
Everything® **Parent's Guide to Raising a Successful Child**
Everything® **Parenting a Teenager Book**
Everything® **Potty Training Book**, $9.95 ($15.95 CAN)
Everything® **Pregnancy Book, 2nd Ed.**
Everything® **Pregnancy Fitness Book**
Everything® **Pregnancy Organizer**, $15.00 ($22.95 CAN)
Everything® **Toddler Book**
Everything® **Tween Book**

PERSONAL FINANCE

Everything® **Budgeting Book**
Everything® **Get Out of Debt Book**
Everything® **Get Rich Book**
Everything® **Homebuying Book, 2nd Ed.**
Everything® **Homeselling Book**
Everything® **Investing Book**
Everything® **Money Book**
Everything® **Mutual Funds Book**
Everything® **Online Investing Book**
Everything® **Personal Finance Book**
Everything® **Personal Finance in Your 20s & 30s Book**
Everything® **Wills & Estate Planning Book**

PETS

Everything® **Cat Book**
Everything® **Dog Book**
Everything® **Dog Training and Tricks Book**
Everything® **Golden Retriever Book**
Everything® **Horse Book**
Everything® **Labrador Retriever Book**
Everything® **Puppy Book**
Everything® **Tropical Fish Book**

All Everything® books are priced at $12.95 or $14.95, unless otherwise stated. Prices subject to change without notice.
Canadian prices range from $11.95–$31.95, and are subject to change without notice.

REFERENCE

Everything® **Astronomy Book**
Everything® **Car Care Book**
Everything® **Christmas Book, $15.00**
  ($21.95 CAN)
Everything® **Classical Mythology Book**
Everything® **Einstein Book**
Everything® **Etiquette Book**
Everything® **Great Thinkers Book**
Everything® **Philosophy Book**
Everything® **Psychology Book**
Everything® **Shakespeare Book**
Everything® **Tall Tales, Legends, &**
  Other Outrageous
  Lies Book
Everything® **Toasts Book**
Everything® **Trivia Book**
Everything® **Weather Book**

RELIGION

Everything® **Angels Book**
Everything® **Bible Book**
Everything® **Buddhism Book**
Everything® **Catholicism Book**
Everything® **Christianity Book**
Everything® **Jewish History &**
  Heritage Book
Everything® **Judaism Book**
Everything® **Prayer Book**
Everything® **Saints Book**
Everything® **Understanding Islam**
  Book
Everything® **World's Religions Book**
Everything® **Zen Book**

SCHOOL & CAREERS

Everything® **After College Book**
Everything® **Alternative Careers Book**
Everything® **College Survival Book**
Everything® **Cover Letter Book**
Everything® **Get-a-Job Book**
Everything® **Hot Careers Book**

Everything® **Job Interview Book**
Everything® **New Teacher Book**
Everything® **Online Job Search Book**
Everything® **Resume Book, 2nd Ed.**
Everything® **Study Book**

SELF-HELP/ RELATIONSHIPS

Everything® **Dating Book**
Everything® **Divorce Book**
Everything® **Great Marriage Book**
Everything® **Great Sex Book**
Everything® **Kama Sutra Book**
Everything® **Romance Book**
Everything® **Self-Esteem Book**
Everything® **Success Book**

SPORTS & FITNESS

Everything® **Body Shaping Book**
Everything® **Fishing Book**
Everything® **Fly-Fishing Book**
Everything® **Golf Book**
Everything® **Golf Instruction Book**
Everything® **Knots Book**
Everything® **Pilates Book**
Everything® **Running Book**
Everything® **Sailing Book, 2nd Ed.**
Everything® **T'ai Chi and QiGong Book**
Everything® **Total Fitness Book**
Everything® **Weight Training Book**
Everything® **Yoga Book**

TRAVEL

Everything® **Family Guide to Hawaii**
Everything® **Guide to Las Vegas**
Everything® **Guide to New England**
Everything® **Guide to New York City**
Everything® **Guide to Washington D.C.**
Everything® **Travel Guide to The Dis-**
  neyland Resort®, Cali-
  fornia Adventure®,

Universal Studios®, and
the Anaheim Area
Everything® **Travel Guide to the Walt**
  Disney World Resort®, Uni-
  versal Studios®, and
  Greater Orlando, 3rd Ed.

WEDDINGS

Everything® **Bachelorette Party Book,**
  $9.95 ($15.95 CAN)
Everything® **Bridesmaid Book, $9.95**
  ($15.95 CAN)
Everything® **Creative Wedding Ideas**
  Book
Everything® **Elopement Book, $9.95**
  ($15.95 CAN)
Everything® **Groom Book**
Everything® **Jewish Wedding Book**
Everything® **Wedding Book, 2nd Ed.**
Everything® **Wedding Checklist,**
  $7.95 ($11.95 CAN)
Everything® **Wedding Etiquette Book,**
  $7.95 ($11.95 CAN)
Everything® **Wedding Organizer,**
  $15.00 ($22.95 CAN)
Everything® **Wedding Shower Book,**
  $7.95 ($12.95 CAN)
Everything® **Wedding Vows Book,**
  $7.95 ($11.95 CAN)
Everything® **Weddings on a Budget**
  Book, $9.95 ($15.95 CAN)

WRITING

Everything® **Creative Writing Book**
Everything® **Get Published Book**
Everything® **Grammar and Style Book**
Everything® **Grant Writing Book**
Everything® **Guide to Writing Chil-**
  dren's Books
Everything® **Screenwriting Book**
Everything® **Writing Well Book**